Handbook of Microbiological Investigations for Laboratory Animal Health

Handbook of Microbiological Investigations for Laboratory Animal Health

J. R. Needham

Division of Comparative Medicine
Clinical Research Centre, Harrow HA1 3UJ, England
Visiting Lecturer, Paddington College, London W2

1979

ACADEMIC PRESS
London · New York · San Francisco
A Subsidiary of Harcourt Brace Jovanovich, Publishers

ACADEMIC PRESS INC. (LONDON) LTD
24–28 Oval Road
London NW1

U.S. Edition published by
ACADEMIC PRESS INC.
111 Fifth Avenue
New York, New York 10003

Needham, J.
Handbook of microbiological investigations
for animal health.
1. Veterinary microbiology—Technique
I. Title
636.089′601′028 QR49 79–40091
ISBN 0–12–515950–1

PRINTED IN GREAT BRITAIN BY
LATIMER TREND & COMPANY LTD
PLYMOUTH

Preface

The control of infectious diseases contributes significantly to the welfare of all animal species and to the successful management of establishments where they are maintained. In the case of laboratory animals, used either for experiments or for the testing of pharmaceutical products, disease control is essential if the objectives of the investigations are to be fulfilled.

The information presented in this book is based principally on microbiological techniques employed at the Clinical Research Centre to complement the animal health and quality control programme. In a programme of this kind it is not possible to include all available laboratory tests and it is recognized that other workers may find it necessary to employ different tests and, possibly, also to modify or discard some of those described here. However, it is hoped that the contents of this volume may provide at least an initial guide for those who wish to establish a similar laboratory.

I would particularly like to thank Dr C. R. Coid and Dr C. J. Green who were responsible for initially establishing the animal health and quality control programmes and for their continual encouragement. Mr J. E. Cooper kindly provided me with advice and carried out the majority of histological examinations described. Finally, I must thank my wife Gina without whose tolerance and help the compilation of this book would have been infinitely more difficult.

June 1979 J. R. NEEDHAM

Contents

List of Figures

List of Plates

List of Tables

1

Introduction

The Animal House at the Clinical Research Centre, Harrow, England, was ready for occupation in late 1970, and the nucleus of scientific staff and animal technicians who had earlier been appointed, moved from temporary accommodation at the National Institute for Medical Research, Mill Hill, England. It was decided that the Division would have a major service commitment to supply and house animals for all other research divisions, as well as the adjoining Northwick Park Hospital, and would also carry out its own research programme and collaborate with other divisions in multi-disciplinary investigations. The service commitment was expected to be the major part of the division's work, correctly as it transpired, for some 30 000 animals are now being held at any given time (Appendix 1). From the outset, it was decided that an animal health and quality control programme should be established. All the work was to be handled within the Division and was the responsibility of a veterinary surgeon and a qualified laboratory technologist, specialized in microbiology. There were several reasons why it was felt essential to have a programme and these are discussed below.

When the Animal House accommodation was finished, animals already included in long term experiments were transferred from other research units to be housed within the Clinical Research Centre (CRC) facility. This clearly introduced the hazard of many species of micro-organisms colonizing the new building, some of them potential pathogens. It was, therefore, decided that priority should be given to the microbiological screening of these animals on arrival at the Centre.

It was considered essential to breed at least 90% of the rodents required by workers in a hysterectomy derived barrier maintained unit. It was anticipated that the issue of animals of known microbiological status would assist the research worker and improve the health status of the animals within the building. However, it was realized that until this unit was producing sufficient numbers, rodents would have to be purchased from commercial laboratory mouse breeders to supply the 150 workers already appointed. This policy exposed the new building to the hazard of microbiological contamination. In an attempt to minimize this risk it was decided that animals would only be purchased from breeders accredited by the Laboratory Animals Centre, Carshalton, Surrey. It was known that few breeders ran their own quality control programmes, so regular health checks on purchased animals were instituted immediately the animals arrived at the Clinical Research Centre.

Some species of farm animal were to be kept at the facility for long term antiserum production, as well as experimental procedures, including major surgery. Each species of animal, whether pigs, calves, sheep or goats would present different disease problems. Enteric, and to a lesser extent respiratory disease, cause the biggest problems in housed farm animals, so it was decided that regular microbiological screening of the animals' faeces would be carried out to detect the introduction of enteric pathogens into the facility.

At least 20 000 animals are in use in experiments at any one time, many of which are long term, some lasting in excess of 2 years. With the expertise available in the Division, it was intended to offer both veterinary and laboratory assistance to research workers. It was considered essential to issue rodents to research workers, that were known to be free from the common pathogens, so that experiments would not be hampered by intercurrent disease. In order to ensure that the animals were of constant microbiological status, it was decided that mice and rats issued from the breeding unit should be regularly examined, probably the most important function of the quality control programme. It was also realized that research workers might encounter health problems in their animals, whilst these were on experiment; therefore the health programme would provide a diagnostic service backed up by veterinary treatment based on the laboratory results. It was known that this service would be required particularly for the larger animals, for instance dogs being used for major surgery, although it has also proved of great value in the diagnosis and control of rodent disease.

Finally, it was decided that the quality control programme should include regular surveillance of the environment within the Animal House. The facility is complex (Appendices 2 and 3), with several specialized areas including a suite for use with infectious agents. It was decided that by testing water, food, autoclave function, staff health and air samples, microbiological contamination would be detected early so that preventative steps could be taken to exclude entry of microorganisms to the animals.

Having decided that a health screening programme was necessary, a closer examination was made of the various areas from which it was thought that specimens should be taken and it was decided that it would be profitable to establish:

(1) Regular microbiological screening of the rodent breeding colony, including the newly established barrier maintained breeding unit.

(2) Microbiological screening of animals purchased from commercial laboratory animal breeders.

(3) Placing of sentinel mice in all rodent holding rooms and subsequent regular microbiological examination.

(4) Pathological examination of any dead animals or those appearing unwell.

(5) Regular examination of faeces from primates and farm animals for enteric pathogens.

(6) Diagnostic service for post-operative infections in large animals.

(7) Monitoring of the environment.

(8) Research projects related to animal health and quality control.

Before formulating any definite details of the microbiological programme a literature search was conducted to see whether any similar programmes were in existence. This revealed a scarcity of reports of health control programmes in animal houses; in fact Izard and Roberts (1960) were the only authors giving details of a laboratory animal health programme. Tuffery (1959, 1962) reported the results of health programmes but dealt mainly with a statistical approach to the subject. Three more general papers were found (Lane-Petter *et al.,* 1955; Seamer and Chesterman, 1967; Tuffery, 1956) but none of these dealt directly with the detailed laboratory investigations of animal health problems. It was decided therefore that the details of the programme would be evolved according to the needs of the work of the Division.

The work recorded in this book was performed over a $2\frac{1}{2}$ year period. Details are recorded of the evolution of the laboratory programme including experiments to devise microbiological techniques necessary for the screening of the mouse colonies and sub-human primates. Experiments were conducted to investigate the treatment of mice infested by ectoparasites, and several experiments were performed to study aspects of the colonization of mice issued from the barrier maintained breeding unit by bacteria. Details are also recorded of the diagnostic service for large animals.

2

Laboratory Techniques Involved in the Health Scheme

Introduction

As the animal health laboratory would be receiving various types of specimens from a wide range of sources, it was decided to categorize these sources before formulating any screening protocol:

Breeding Colony

It was considered vital that any animals showing signs of clinical illness in the rodent breeding colony should be examined. Animals were sent to the laboratory by the staff running the breeding programmes.

Routine Screen

This was anticipated to be the largest section and included the sampling of faeces from monkeys and farm animals, random microbiological checks on stock animals and rodents in the breeding unit, autoclave testing and control of staff health.

Sentinel Mice

In order that a constant check of the microbiological status of various areas within the Animal House could be made, mice issued from the barrier unit were placed within these areas, and were sampled at regular intervals.

Research Workers

At the request of research workers, samples were taken from animals with signs of clinical illness or they were collected in an effort to resolve unexpected experimental results.

Having categorized the main areas of investigation, thought was given to the types of specimens to be examined. These ranged from live animals to wound swabs. No firm idea of the numbers could be obtained and therefore the sample size was to be decided as each occasion arose and will be discussed in each appropriate section.

Before any protocols were drawn up, standard text books were consulted to determine whether suitable methods for the examination of specimens existed. It was felt reasonable to rely to a great extent on standard medical microbiological techniques. Veterinary pathology text books such as Davies (1962) and Boddie (1962) described animal diseases but usually gave little specific information on the exact procedures adopted for their laboratory diagnosis. The Laboratory Animals Centre was consulted and provided basic information which was helpful in formulating some procedures.

A large proportion of the work involved in the animal screening programme was concerned with the *post mortem* examination of the whole animal, so a scheme was designed which it was hoped would ensure that the fullest possible pathological examination was carried out on each animal. This scheme was to cover the major branches of pathology, namely bacteriology, virology, mycoplasmology, parasitology and histopathology. Whenever the need arose, experiments were performed in the hope of designing new techniques or improving those existing and these will be reported in Chapter 3.

Materials and Methods

Bacteriology

The primary medium used for the isolation of bacteria from all sites, excluding faeces, was blood agar. Selenite F and deoxycholate citrate agar were used for the screening of faeces as recommended by Blackmore and Hill (1972a). All plates were incubated at 37°C aerobically. If there was scanty or no growth after 18 h the plates were incubated for a further 24 h. Other media were used if indicated. The choice of medium and cultural method varied according to the nature of the lesion; for example, Loefflers serum agar slopes were used to culture eye swabs, and specimens from liver or kidney lesions were cultured anaerobically.

Initially, the lungs of each animal were examined using the lung wash fluid but this was later superceded by a cut lung surface technique (see Chapter 3).

Mycoplasmology

Specimens were obtained from throats and lungs and were first cultured in mycoplasma broth as described by Chanock *et al.* (1962), followed by culture on solid medium.

Broth medium was divided into 1·8 ml aliquots in small glass vials. The throat swab was placed in broth immediately it was taken and allowed to soak for 1 min. As much broth as possible was expressed from the swab and dilutions of 10^{-1} to 10^{-3} were made. All four broths were then incubated as described below.

Recovery of mycoplasmas from the lungs was attempted by a perfusion technique (Taylor-Robinson *et al.,* 1972). The fluid used was mycoplasma basal broth (Difco Laboratories, West Molesey, Surrey) and 0·2 ml of the recovered fluid was added to 1·8 ml of broth giving an initial dilution of 10^{-1}. Further dilutions of 10^{-2} and 10^{-3} were made. All broths were incubated at 37°C for up to 4 weeks and were inspected for colour change (red to yellow) every 2 days; any showing a colour change were repassaged into broth and plated out on to solid mycoplasma medium (Difco Laboratories, West Molesey, Surrey), supplemented with horse serum, yeast extract and glucose. This was incubated at 37°C for 7 days in an atmosphere of 5% carbon dioxide and 95% nitrogen. However, if no colour change was noted in the broth medium, samples were plated out on to solid medium after 2 weeks had elapsed, and this was repeated after a further 2 weeks. No attempt was made to type any mycoplasmas isolated.

Parasitology

Each rodent submitted for examination was carefully examined for ectoparasites, with particular reference to the mange mites *Myobia musculi* and *Myocoptes musculinus*. Caecal contents were subjected to macroscopic examination for the presence of worms. Wet preparations of faeces were microscopically examined for the presence of ova of *Hymenolepis nana* and *Syphacia obvelata*, the oocysts of *Eimeria falciformis* and the protozoa *Hexamita muris* and *Giardia muris*. Flotation and concentration techniques were not used.

Virology

The possible presence of virus infections in animals was mainly examined by serological methods although in the case of Ectromelia (mouse pox) animal inoculation was used as the reputedly more reliable method. This test has now been superceded by a serological method (Carthew and Verstraete, 1978).

Serology

Two serological tests were regularly performed as part of the screening protocol. Both were haemagglutination inhibition (HI) tests and these were used for evidence of infection by Sendai virus and pneumonia virus of mice (PVM). The tests will be described in detail in Chapter 3.

Animal Inoculation

This method was used to check the mouse stock for the presence of Ectromelia virus. Batches of six mice varying in age between 4 and 10 weeks, were placed in an exhaust ventilated isolator and lightly anaesthetized with ether. Calf lymph vaccinia vaccine was applied to a scarified area at the base of the tail and the mice were allowed to recover from the anaesthetic within the isolator and remain there throughout the test. The vaccinated area was viewed daily for 5 days by which time a reaction was seen; reddening and swelling took place in those animals with no history of Ectromelia infection.

Histopathology

During the first few months of the health scheme, samples of liver, kidney, spleen and lungs were taken routinely from animals under examination, but this was later reduced so that specimens were only collected from organs with obvious lesions present at autopsy.

All specimens were fixed in 10% formal saline prior to embedding in paraffin wax and staining with Coles haematoxylin and eosin. The prepared slides were then viewed by the veterinary pathologist. The results obtained were used as confirmation of microbiological results and will not, therefore, be reported in detail.

Post-mortem Examination of Rodents (Figure 1)

Whenever possible live animals were submitted for pathological examination. However, in cases where dead or moribund animals were presented, these were examined as fully as practicable and the limitations accepted by the pathologist.

The animals were killed by an overdose of sodium pentobarbitone ("Sagatal", May and Baker Ltd, Dagenham, Kent) administered by intraperitoneal injection. Once unconscious, the skin and fur were examined under a ×20 dissecting microscope for the presence of ectoparasites. Careful attention was paid to the head, particularly the muzzle and eyelids.

The animals were secured in dorsal recumbency on a cork board and placed under a protective clean air hood. This was operated with the air filtration unit switched off, as it was felt that the animal was suitably protected from contamination. A bunsen burner was provided for the sterilization of instruments. The skin was opened along the mid line, from the mandible to the pubis. Blood was collected from the right axilla, after severing the jugular vein and carotid artery. The mouth was opened wide by grasping the mandible and tongue using a pair of forceps and a throat swab was collected utilizing a nasopharyngeal swab (Calgiswab ref. 65-150-15, A. R. Horwell, Kilburn High Road, London) and this was rubbed on to a blood agar plate. A second swab was taken for mycoplasmology and treated as described earlier in this chapter. Care was taken to ensure that the swab did not touch the tongue or teeth.

After the throat swabs had been taken, the trachea was exposed by dissecting the overlying muscles and was ligated approximately half way between the larynx and the bronchial bifurcation. (Figs 2, 3 and 4.) Mycoplasma basal broth was introduced into the trachea, using a 26 g needle and 1 ml syringe, so that both lungs were perfused. After 15 s, to allow for fluid distribution within the lungs, as much of the fluid was

Discipline	Specimen	Test
Bacteriology	Throat swab	Blood agar 24 and 48 hours.
	Cut lung surface	Blood agar 24 and 48 hours.
	Caecum	Desoxycholate Citrate Agar 24 hours.
		Selenite F 24 hours-Desoxycholate Citrate Agar 24 hours.
Mycoplasmology	Throat swab	Liquid medium, plate 2weeks and 4 weeks.
	Lung wash	Same as throat swab.
Virology	Animal inoculation	Ectromelia
	Serology	Sendai (Haemagglutination Inhibition)
		Mouse hepatitis (Complement fixation test)
		Pneumonia virus of mice (Haemagglutination Inhibition)
		Reo III (Haemagglutination Inhibition)
		Polyoma (Haemagglutination Inhibition)
Parasitology	Skin	Microscopical examination for ectoparasites.
	Gut	Jejunum, Ileum, Caecum (Macroscopic examination-wet prep.)
Histology	Lungs	Haematoxylin and Eosin
	Liver	
	Spleen	
	Kidneys	

Fig. 1. Scheme for *post mortem* examination of animals.

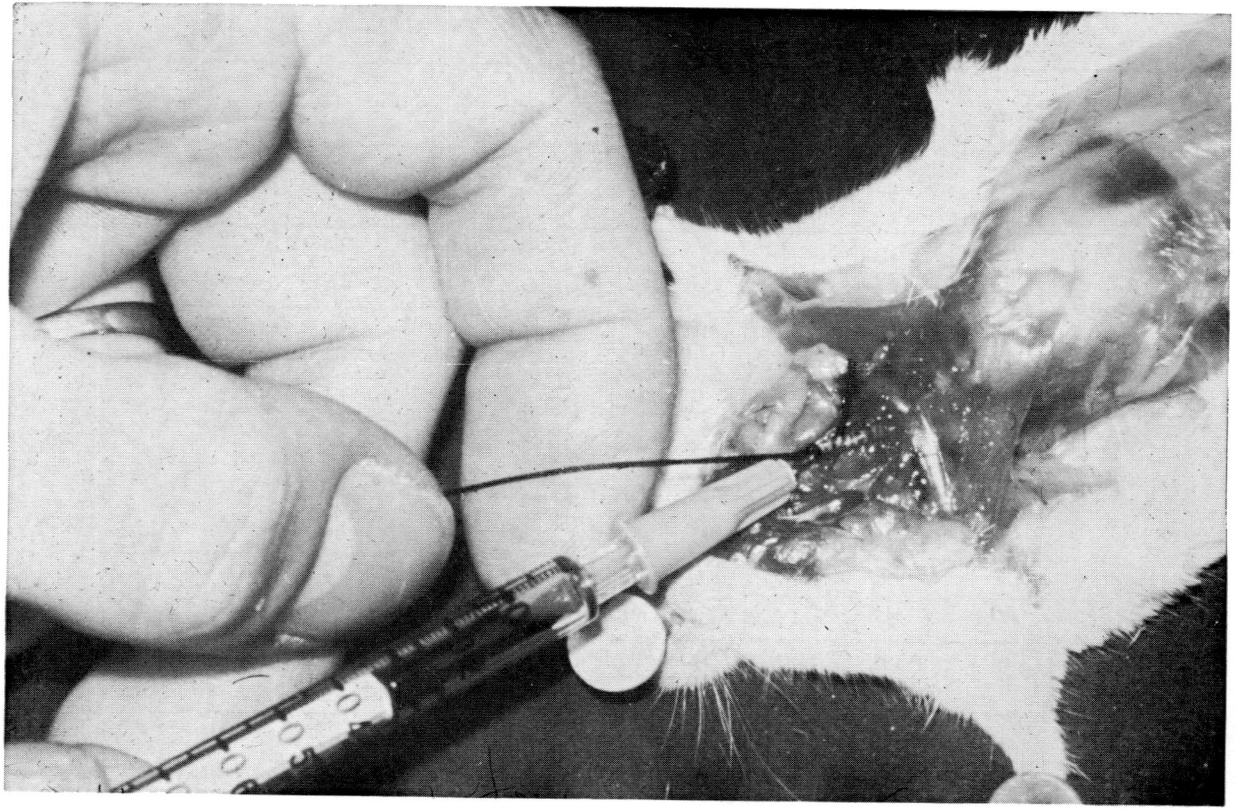

Fig. 2. Mouse lung wash technique.

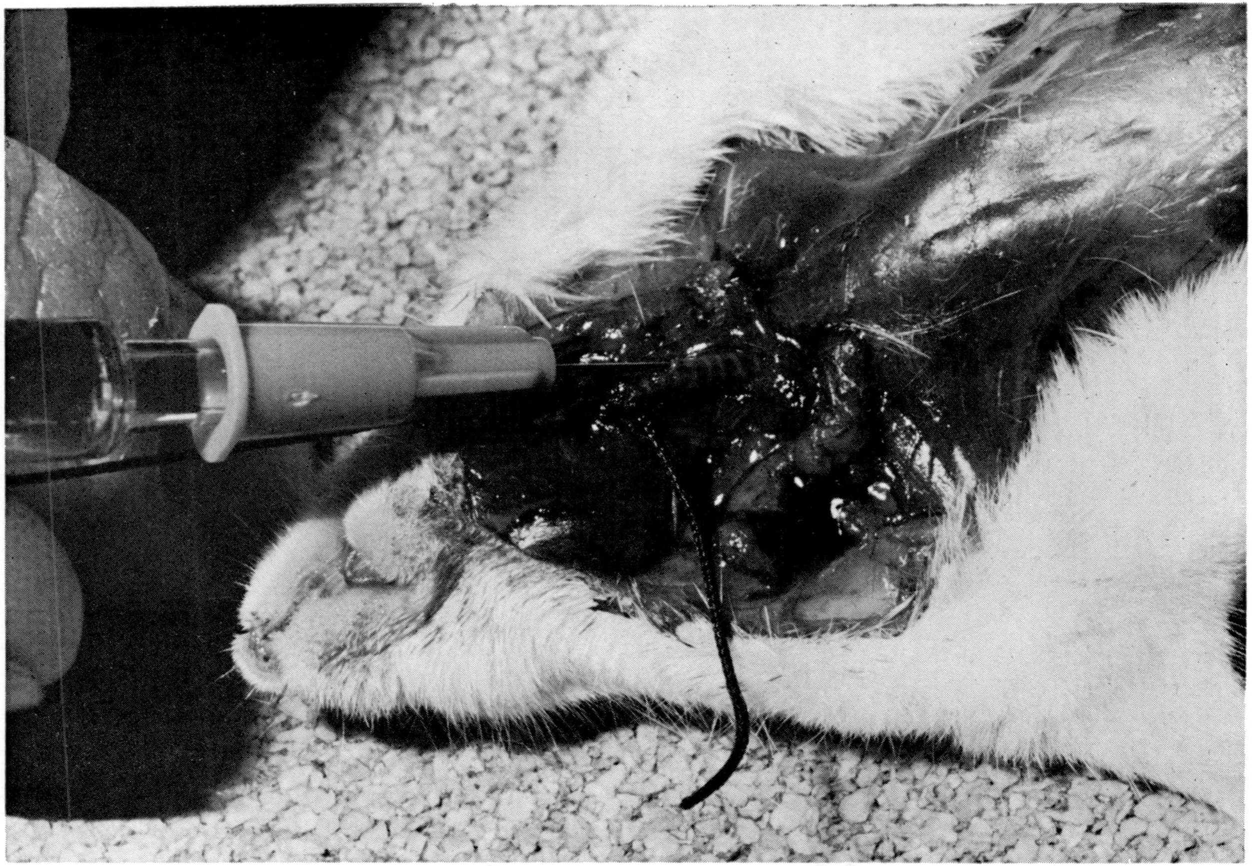

Fig. 3. Mouse lung wash technique.

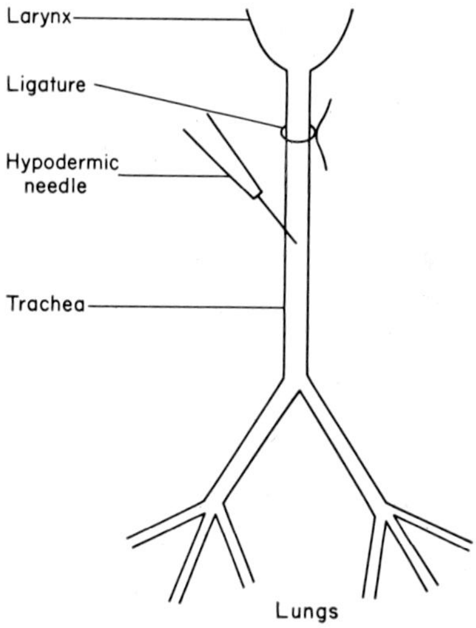

Fig. 4. Mouse lung wash technique.

recovered as possible and 0·2 ml was added to mycoplasma broth and treated as already described. This technique was an adaptation of a method described by Taylor-Robinson *et al.* (1972). The volume of fluid used for the lung wash depended on the size of the animal.

Initially, the lung wash fluid was examined bacteriologically, but, this method was superceded by the cut surface technique as this was shown, by experiment (see Chapter 3), to yield a higher recovery rate. The thorax of the animal was opened with sterile instruments and the lungs examined for lesions. The diaphragmatic lobe was cut with a pair of scissors which had been soaked in alcohol and flamed and the free portion of the lobe was rubbed on to a blood agar plate in such a way that only the freshly cut surface had contact with the plate. Finally, the abdominal cavity was opened and a visual examination of all organs made. If no abnormalities or lesions were present the caecum was removed and the contents expressed into a dish. A portion was placed on to a deoxycholate citrate agar plate (DCA) which was incubated at 37°C for up to 48 h. Another portion was placed in selenite F medium, which was incubated for 72 h with sub-cultures being made on DCA at 24 and 72 h (Chattopadhyay and Pilford, 1976).

If at any stage of the examination lesions were observed, the affected area of the organ was subjected to bacteriological culture and a sample of tissue placed in 10% formal saline prior to histopathological examination.

Miscellaneous Samples

Blood Cultures

Samples of blood (10 ml) from dogs were drawn aseptically from the brachiocephalic vein and distributed into three blood culture bottles containing 7 ml of nutrient broth with 0·05% liquoid (sodium polyanethol sulphonate). If growth was observed after incubation at 37°C, sub-cultures were made on to blood agar plates which were incubated aerobically and anaerobically, but if not, sub-cultures were made at 7 and 14 days.

Wound Swabs and Exudates

These specimens were cultured on two blood agar plates, one incubated aerobically, the other anaerobically. A portion of the specimen, or the complete swab, was also placed in Robertson's cooked meat medium. After 48 h incubation, or earlier if growth was visible, sub-cultures were made on to blood agar.

Faeces

Faecal samples from monkeys, dogs and farm animals were obtained as fresh as possible (Needham, 1977). Samples were collected on to a spoon contained in a sterile universal bottle (Sterilin Ltd, Teddington, Middlesex). The faeces were plated on to deoxycholate citrate agar and inoculated in to selenite F.

Nasal Swabs

Nasal swabs were taken from all staff concerned with the rodent barrier maintained breeding unit at monthly intervals. The swabs were plated on to blood agar and chocolate agar plates which were incubated aerobically at 37°C for 18 h. Coagulase positive staphylococci were sent to the Central Public Health Laboratory, Colindale, for phage typing.

3

Development of New Laboratory Techniques

Introduction

During the first weeks of the animal health programme, it was realized that three laboratory techniques were not yielding satisfactory results: (a) the perfusion technique for the bacteriological examination of lungs, (b) the identification of staphylococci using the coagulase test and the production of deoxyribonuclease, and (c) the haemagglutination inhibition test for evidence of infection with Sendai virus and pneumonia virus of mice.

It was decided that each of these three tests must be investigated and, where necessary, new protocols evolved.

Comparison of Lung Wash and Cut Lung Surface Techniques

Introduction

The knowledge of the microbiological status of the lungs was considered important due to the high incidence of respiratory disease amongst rodent populations. The sampling technique had to be easy to carry out, quick, and free from the risk of contamination. For these reasons it was decided to make use of the lung wash fluid recovered for mycoplasmology.

However, it became apparent that this method was not suitable for the isolation of bacteria as very few organisms were recovered, even though many samples were taken from cases of respiratory disease, with obvious lung lesions.

Experiments were set up to compare the number of bacterial isolates obtained from mice lungs when a straightforward cut lung surface technique was used as an alternative to washing out the lungs.

Materials and Methods

Animals

The mice used were 8-week-old TO/Crc strain of either sex, issued from the barrier maintained breeding unit. Immediately on issue, the mice were placed in an isolator where they were left for the duration of the experiment. Food and water were supplied *ad libatum.*

Organism

The organism used was *Pasteurella pneumotropica,* originally obtained from a mouse throat. It was identified according to Cowan and Steel (1966) and agglutinated with specific antiserum supplied by the Laboratory Animals Centre, Carshalton, Surrey. A culture was grown on blood agar for 18 h and a suspension made in sterile phosphate buffered saline.

Methods

Experiment 1

Sixty male mice were intranasally inoculated with approximately 1×10^3 organisms, whilst under light ether anaesthesia. On day 3 post inoculation, 20 mice were removed for examination. The animals were killed with an overdose of sodium pentobarbitone injected intraperitoneally and the lungs were washed, as already described in Chapter 2, using peptone water as the wash medium. 0·1 ml of the wash medium was plated on to a blood agar plate which was incubated overnight at 37°C. The lungs were removed and the cut surface of one lobe rubbed on to a blood agar plate. After incubation, all plates were read qualitatively for the presence of *Pasteurella pneumotropica*. 20 mice were also examined on day 4 and a further 20 on day 7 post inoculation.

Experiment 2 was carried out in a similar way but using mycoplasma basal broth without crystal violet (Difco Laboratories, West Molesey, Surrey) as the wash fluid, and in experiment 3, brain heart infusion broth was used.

The three experiments were repeated (experiments 4–6) with female, 8-week-old TO/Crc mice and finally the experiments were repeated (experiments 7–9) inoculating 36 female mice and 36 male mice simultaneously for each experiment.

Results

The results are summarized in Table 1; showing that approximately two isolates were obtained from cut lung surfaces for every one from a lung wash. When the results were examined for individual experiments (experiments 1–9) as shown in Tables 2, 3 and 4, the 2:1 ratio was also found. This ratio was not dependent on the day post inoculation that the mouse was examined or on the wash medium used. However, female mice yielded less isolates than male mice.

Table 1

Experiments 1–9: number of isolates of *Pasteurella pneumotropica* obtained from mice following intranasal inoculation

	Number positive	
Medium	Cut lung	Lung perfusion
Peptone water	91/172	47/172
Mycoplasma broth	67/172	30/172
Brain heart infusion broth	89/172	48/172

Table 2

Experiments 1–3: number of isolates of *Pasteurella pneumotropica* obtained from 8-week-old male mice following intranasal inoculation

Day post inoculation	Medium	Number positive	
		Cut lung	Lung perfusion
Day 3	PEP	15/20	11/20
	PPLO	10/20	6/20
	BHI	12/20	4/20
Day 4	PEP	15/20	9/20
	PPLO	11/20	6/20
	BHI	12/20	8/20
Day 7	PEP	12/20	8/20
	PPLO	9/20	6/20
	BHI	12/20	8/20

PEP, peptone water, Experiment 1; PPLO, mycoplasma broth, Experiment 2; BHI, brain heart infusion broth, Experiment 3.

Table 3

Experiments 4–6: number of isolates of *Pasteurella pneumotropica* obtained from 8-week-old female mice following intranasal inoculation

Day post inoculation	Medium	Number positive	
		Cut lung	Lung perfusion
Day 3	PEP	5/20	0/20
	PPLO	5/20	2/20
	BHI	10/20	6/20
Day 4	PEP	5/20	2/20
	PPLO	5/20	2/20
	BHI	7/20	2/20
Day 7	PEP	7/20	3/20
	PPLO	4/20	3/20
	BHI	6/20	6/20

PEP, peptone water, Experiment 4; PPLO, mycoplasma broth, Experiment 5; BHI, brain heart infusion broth, Experiment 6.

Table 4

Experiments 7–9: number of isolates of *Pasteurella pneumotropica* obtained from 8-week-old male and female mice inoculated intranasally

		Number positive			
		Male		Female	
Day post inoculation	Medium	Cut lung	Lung perfusion	Cut lung	Lung perfusion
	PEP	12/12	5/12	2/12	1/12
Day 3	PPLO	5/12	1/12	3/12	1/12
	BHI	7/12	4/12	2/12	3/12
	PEP	8/12	4/12	2/12	2/12
Day 4	PPLO	6/12	2/12	3/12	0/12
	BHI	12/12	4/12	2/12	1/12
	PEP	5/12	2/12	3/12	0/12
Day 7	PPLO	4/12	1/12	2/12	0/12
	BHI	5/12	1/12	3/12	1/12

PEP, peptone water, Experiment 7; PPLO, mycoplasma broth, Experiment 8; BHI, brain heart infusion broth, Experiment 9.

Discussion

In a large animal facility it is essential that respiratory infections are speedily diagnosed and hence recovery techniques must be evolved with this object in mind.

The experiments showed that a cut lung surface technique doubles the chance of recovery of *Pasteurella pneumotropica,* compared with the lung perfusion technique.

The failure of the lung perfusion technique was not entirely unexpected as it had been designed for the recovery of mycoplasmas from the respiratory tract (Taylor-Robinson *et al.,* 1972). These agents are found on the surface of the cells lining the upper respiratory tract and are therefore easily removed by perfusion. Bacteria, however, are more often found within the lung tissue as foci of infection, frequently as abscesses and therefore less likely to be dislodged by a wash-out procedure. On the other hand a cut surface technique will be more successful in locating the foci of infection and recovery of the organisms effected by direct contact.

With any technique it is essential that suspected cases are detected as soon as possible. In the early stages of infection the organisms are more likely to be recovered. Abscesses of long standing may become calcified and in this state are frequently sterile.

The cut surface technique also satisfied other requirements. It was both a quick and a simple procedure. By the observance of aseptic techniques no contamination occurred during the examination of the 516 mice involved in the experiments, as judged by the absence of other species of organisms on the blood agar plates. Using this method it was possible to obtain preliminary diagnosis after overnight incubation. This was an advantage over a method reported by Verstraete (1973) utilizing broth cultures of rodent lung, which required 48 h to obtain a diagnosis.

The experiment designed to study the effect of different media did not appear to show any marked difference. With all media, the cut surface technique resulted in a higher recovery rate. Mycoplasma broth yielded the lowest recovery rate, although still 2:1 in favour of the cut surface technique. No explanation could be found for the drop in the level of recovery, but it was presumed that this was due to a variation in the susceptibility of the mice to the infecting organism. Unfortunately, it was not practicable to carry out all the experiments on one batch of mice.

It was concluded that the cut lung surface technique gave a high rate of bacterial isolation.

Differentiation of Staphylococci: Comparison of the Correlation Between the Coagulase Test and Deoxyribonuclease Test

Introduction

The identification of staphylococci has been of importance to medical and veterinary bacteriologists for many years. *Staphylococcus aureus* is generally differentiated from *Staphylococcus epidermidis* by its ability to produce the enzymes coagulase and deoxyribonuclease and their production is accepted as an indication of the potential pathogenicity of these organisms. It has been shown that there is correlation between the coagulase test and deoxyribonuclease test when applied to staphylococci from human sources (Jacobs *et al.*, 1964: Jarvis and Wynne, 1969: Brandish and Willis, 1970), but this correlation has not been demonstrated using staphylococci isolated from animals. Furthermore, it has been shown that the production of deoxyribonuclease by staphylococci from human patients may be detected after 4 h (Stickler, 1970).

Staphylococci were isolated from a variety of sources, the greatest number being obtained from animals in the barrier maintained breeding unit; random sampling of the mice and rats from this unit yielded staphylococcal isolates from the throats as well as from abscesses, eyes, ears and lungs. Isolates were also obtained from conventionally maintained mice. Swabs were examined from surgical wounds of dogs following severe orthopaedic interference and from specimens taken at *post mortem* examination of these dogs. Staphylococci were frequently isolated, particularly from animals kept on immuno-suppressant drugs. Finally, isolates of the organism were also obtained from settle plates placed in the experimental animal operating theatre complex as part of the environmental control programme.

Staphylococci were identified and differentiated using colonial morphology and pigment, Gram staining reaction, the tube coagulase test and the production of deoxyribonuclease.

It was decided to see whether a close correlation could be obtained between the coagulase test and the deoxyribonuclease test using staphylococci from non-human sources and whether early detection of deoxyribonuclease production was possible. A preliminary report was published (Needham, 1974).

Materials and Methods

Organisms

The staphylococci studied (Table 5) were isolated from post operative wound lesions of dogs, from throat swabs, skin and abscesses of mice and rats and from other animals including rabbits, guinea-pigs, monkeys and ferrets. They were also isolated from routine air sampling settle plates placed at 16 sites within the operating theatre complex. The Oxford staphylococcus was used as a positive control and a strain of *Staphylococcus epidermidis* as a negative control for the coagulase and deoxyribonuclease tests.

Table 5

Number of staphylococci studied

Source	Canine	Mice	Rats	Other animals	Operating theatres
Number	39	740	155	37	102

Coagulase test

All staphylococci isolated were subjected to the tube test (Fisk, 1940) using coagulase plasma (Difco Laboratories, West Molesey, Surrey).

Deoxyribonuclease test

The staphylococci were isolated on blood agar plates and subsequently spot inoculated on to DNase agar (Oxoid Ltd, Basingstoke, Hants.). Each 9 cm plate contained 15 cm^3 of agar. The plates were developed using 1·5 N hydrochloric acid.

In the initial trial, using the first 20 coagulase positive staphylococci isolated from mouse throat swabs, each organism was inoculated on to two DNase agar plates. One plate was developed after 8 h incubation and the other after 18 h.

In a later trial, 20 coagulase positive staphylococci isolated from murine abscesses, were each inoculated on to three DNase agar plates. One plate was developed after 4 h incubation, one after 8 h and the last after 18 h. Subsequently all plates involved in this trial were developed after 18 h incubation.

Results

It was noted with the first isolates of murine staphylococci, obtained mainly from throat swabs, that the clotting time of the coagulase plasma was, in 90% of cases, in excess of 6 h. Therefore on the initial trial, samples were incubated for either 8 or 18 h.

At 8 h the Oxford staphylococcus gave a clear zone of approximately 6 mm surrounding the macro colony on the DNase plate. However,

Table 6

Results of initial deoxyribonuclease trial

Source	Tube coagulase	Deoxyribonuclease 8 h incubation	Deoxyribonuclease 18 h incubation
Mouse throat swabs	20/20	3/20	20/20

the 20 staphylococci forming the initial trial gave zones of 2–3 mm or less after 8 h incubation, although after 18 h, zone sizes of up to 6 mm were obtained. Using this length of time of incubation and applying a zone size of 6 mm, the test then correlated with the coagulase test (Table 6).

Later it was found that staphylococci isolated from murine abscesses clotted coagulase plasma in less than 6 h, in some cases as short as 3 h. A second trial showed that it was still necessary to incubate the deoxyribonuclease test for 18 h to achieve correlation with the coagulase test (Table 7). Staphylococci from abscesses did not produce detectable deoxyribonuclease within 4 h and the correlation at 8 h was only slightly improved over the initial trial.

Table 7

Results of second deoxyribonuclease trial

Source	Tube coagulase	Deoxyribonuclease 4 h incubation	8 h incubation	18 h incubation
Mouse abscesses	20/20	2/20	5/20	20/20

A total of 1073 isolates of staphylococci were tested in the survey and correlation between the two tests was achieved with 1066 isolates (99%) (Table 8). The two canine, tube coagulase negative deoxyribonuclease positive staphylococci were both found to be coagulase positive when tested with canine plasma. All other non-correlating isolates were tested with homologous plasma but they were found to remain coagulase negative.

Discussion

The differentiation of staphylococci by the two tests has been used by medical bacteriologists for some years. It is claimed that the tests may be used to obtain a result within 4 h of setting up and it was therefore thought worthy of investigation when this could not be achieved in this time with staphylococci from animal sources.

The first observation noted was that the staphylococci appeared to grow slower than their human counterparts. Plasma coagulated only after at least 6 h incubation and in many cases only after overnight incubation.

Table 8

Distribution of coagulase activity and deoxyribonuclease production after 18 h incubation

Source	Number	Tube coagulase	Deoxyribonuclease
Dogs	28	+	+
	2	—	+
	9	—	—
Mice	614	+	+
	3	—	+
	123	—	—
Rats	140	+	+
	2	—	+
	13	—	—
Other animals	25	+	+
	12	—	—
Operating theatre complex	27	+	+
	75	—	—

When isolates of *Staphylococcus aureus* from murine abscesses were tested, the coagulation time was found to be shorter, until in some cases coagulation was seen within 3 h. This was thought to indicate increased virulence of the organism as manifested by the appearance at that time of many abscesses.

The two experiments carried out to detect early formation of deoxyribonuclease were incubated for periods based on the time taken for coagulation of plasma to occur. In the first experiment no correlation was achieved between the two tests after 8 h, even though the plasma coagulated. With the virulent staphylococci in the second trial, no deoxyribonuclease was produced as early as 4 h and only slightly better correlation was achieved after 8 h. However, consistent agreement between the two tests was achieved if incubation was carried out for 18 h.

The early detection of deoxyribonuclease production was also hindered by the zone size surrounding the macro colony. With the zone size of only 2–3 mm found after 8 h incubation, interpretation of the result varied with the member of personnel reading the test. However, by 18 h the zone size was at least 6 mm and hence not subject to variable interpretation.

Applying the criteria of 18 h incubation and a 6 mm zone size, good correlation was found between the two tests (Table 8). A small number of *Staphylococcus epidermidis* were found to be deoxyribonuclease producing. Other workers (Jacobs *et al.*, 1964; Jarvis *et al.*, 1969) have also encountered deoxyribonuclease producing *Staphylococcus epidermidis*. The two canine staphylococci that were coagulase negative with commercial plasma were found to coagulate canine plasma. The commercial product is usually harvested from rabbits and it is known that canine *Staphylococcus aureus* does not always coagulate rabbit plasma (Parker, 1974). Subsequent to this finding all coagulase negative isolates were tested with homologous plasma.

It was concluded that close correlation was achieved between the coagulase test and deoxyribonuclease test when incubation was carried out for 18 h, but not at shorter periods.

Haemagglutination Inhibition Test for Sendai Virus

Introduction

At the commencement of this study a haemagglutination inhibition (HI) test was in use for the detection of antibodies to Sendai virus, having been recommended by Blackmore *et al.* (1972b).

However, the test was found to give variable results when assayed against positive control antisera of known titre and it was decided to seek an alternative method. Heath (1971) had already reported a technique which was claimed to give reproducible results so it was decided to copy this and compare it with the HI test already in use.

Materials and Methods

Test in use at the Clinical Research Centre for Sendai Virus: Hereafter Referred to as the CRC Test

The test was divided into two parts for the purposes of this assay: the preparation of sera and titration of the antigen in one part and the actual test in the other.

The sera to be tested were treated for the removal of non-specific agglutinins by adding four parts of receptor destroying enzyme (RDE) (Wellcome Reagents Ltd, Beckenham, Kent) to one part of serum. This mixture was incubated at 37°C overnight followed by inactivation at 56°C for 30 min.

The virus antigen was prepared by inoculating the allantoic cavity of 12-day-old embryonated chicken eggs and incubating at 37°C for 48 h. The allantoic fluid was harvested and stored as 1 ml aliquots at −70°C. The antigen was titrated by double diluting 0·25 ml with phosphate buffered saline to give dilutions of 1/2 to 1/4096. Chicken erythrocytes at a dilution of 0·5% were added and, after mixing, the plate was left at room temperature for 1 h (25°C). The end point of the titration was taken as that dilution showing 50% haemagglutination and this dilution was considered to be 1 HA unit.

The sera to be tested were double diluted from 1/5 to 1/5120 using Microtitre apparatus. A standard volume of 0·025 ml was used. Sendai virus was added to all wells at a dilution of 4 HA units and the plates were left for 1 h at room temperature. 0·5% chicken erythrocytes were added to each well as before and the plate was incubated for a further 1 h at room temperature. The titre of the serum was taken as the dilution showing 50% haemagglutination.

The test was controlled with a positive and a negative serum and erythrocyte controls.

The Heath Test (1971)

The test was again divided into two parts; the treatment of sera and the titration of antigen in one part and the actual test forming the second part.

The sera were treated for the removal of non-specific agglutinins. A 1/8 dilution of each serum was made with a 3% suspension of chicken erythrocytes. The sera were then left at 4°C overnight, after which the supernatant fluid was removed and used for testing.

The virus antigen was prepared in embryonated chicken eggs by the method used at the CRC. The harvested allantoic fluid was stored at 4°C with the addition of 0·001% methiolate solution. When required for use, the antigen was titrated by the CRC technique.

Doubling dilutions of each sera were made using Microtitre apparatus and a standard volume of 0·05 ml, each serum being tested in duplicate. Virus was added to all wells at a dilution of 4 HA units and left for 45 min at room temperature. After this incubation period, one volume of 0·5% chicken erythrocytes were added to each well. The plates were mixed thoroughly and left at room temperature for 30 min. Each serum titration was then read and the end point taken as the highest dilution showing a complete button of cells.

Controls were set up using three positive control sera of differing titre, a negative serum and cell controls.

Due to the fundamental differences between the two techniques it was decided to fully investigate them and experiments were performed to compare their reproducibility.

An initial experiment (experiment 1) was set up utilizing 12 murine sera. Each serum was subjected to three separate tests, (a) the Heath test, (b) the Heath test employing reagents produced by the author and (c) the standard CRC test.

Experiment 2 examined the various methods available for the removal of non-specific inhibitors from sera. In Test 1 untreated sera were used. Test 2 utilized receptor destroying enzyme (RDE) treated sera and Test 3 utilized sera treated by RDE and 3% chicken erythrocytes. After treatment, sera were tested by the Heath test.

During these experiments difficulty was experienced due to a degree of haemolysis of the chicken erythrocytes. Each week at the Clinical Research Centre a batch of 8-week-old Light Sussex chickens was exsanguinated and blood was collected with heparin as anticoagulant. The blood was washed three times with saline prior to dilution to 0·5%. The blood used by Heath was derived from a different source. It was obtained from adult chickens kept by a commercial laboratory where the blood was collected into Alsever's solution. It was known that Heath, using these cells, did not experience haemolysis and it was decided to conduct an experiment (experiment 3) using blood collected from adult Rhode Island Red chickens kept by the author at Harrow, and compare the results with those obtained using fowl cells supplied by Heath. The sera were tested in duplicate giving their titre with each source of fowl cells.

Following these experiments regular testing was commenced using the Heath test with erythrocytes obtained from adult Rhode Island Red chickens.

Results

Experiment 1, designed to compare the Heath test and the CRC test showed poor correlation with only 7/12 results agreeing, although when the same sera were compared using the Heath test with CRC reagents, better correlation was achieved with 11/12 results agreeing (Table 9). Following this experiment the removal of non-specific agglutinins was compared using receptor destroying enzyme (RDE) in one aliquot; RDE and erythrocytes in another, and then comparing both with untreated aliquots (experiment 2). The Heath test was used but no results were obtained due to extensive haemolysis. Repeat tests were subject to the same extensive haemolysis. It was found that this could be eliminated

Table 9

Titres of murine serum tested by three methods

	Heath test		
Reference	Heath reagents	CRC reagents	CRC test
KO3	1/128	1/320	1/1280
HN7	1/16	1/16	1/1280
JXB	1/384	1/512	1/320
JY3	1/16	1/16	1/10
HPE	1/64	1/16	1/1280
JL6	1/24	1/16	1/80
KMB	1/8	1/16	1/1280
JLA	1/8	1/16	1/10
KN5	1/8	1/16	1/320
JW1	1/8	1/16	1/40
KN2	1/16	1/16	1/1280
KN4	1/8	1/16	1/320

Interpretation of titres: Heath test: 1/8, no exposure to infection; 1/16, possible exposure to infection; 1/32 and greater, exposure to infection.
Clinical Research Centre test: 1/10, no exposure to infection; 1/20, possible exposure to infection; 1/40 and greater, exposure to infection.

by using erythrocytes obtained from Rhode Island Red chickens. These were used in experiment 3 but it was found that reproducible results could not be obtained using the CRC test. It was therefore decided to discontinue work with the CRC test and to use exclusively the Heath test.

Discussion

The two techniques detailed were fundamentally different and hence it was obvious that experiments would have to be carried out in order that selection of the most suitable technique could be made.

Experiment 1 was a simple investigation involving the testing of 12 sera by both techniques. This showed that only seven of the results obtained were comparable and that the Heath test with CRC reagents did not yield any greater correlation.

A close examination of both techniques yielded some possible causes of discrepancy. First, the method of interpretation of the end point was different. In the Heath test the end point was the highest dilution showing a button of red cells, whereas the CRC test used a 50% haemagglutination end point. This meant that a lower titre would be obtained by the Heath test as a button of cells must occur at a lower dilution than the 50% end point. Therefore, a weakly positive serum in the CRC test would appear negative by the Heath test. The second difference was the treatment of sera for the removal of non-specific agglutinins. The CRC test involved the use of receptor destroying enzyme with heat inactivation. It has been shown that murine antibodies to Sendai virus are heat labile (Fernando and Heath, 1971a). Therefore heat inactivation of sera is likely to be detrimental, particularly when applied to weakly positive sera, giving false negative results. The same authors have shown that for the most efficient removal of non-specific agglutinins, potassium iodate should be used (Fernando and Heath, 1971b). However, the use of 3% chicken erythrocytes will also achieve the same result and erythrocytes are therefore used for their convenience. Another source of difference between the tests was the accuracy of the dilution of sera. The Heath test used volumes of 0·05 ml which was double that used in the CRC method. Furthermore, each serum in the Heath test was titrated in duplicate, thus eliminating error when making dilutions and adding reagents, and also the test was strictly controlled using three positive sera of different titres.

During experiment 2, designed to examine the methods of removal of non-specific agglutinins, extensive haemolysis rendered every test unreadable. It was realized that the diluent was not at fault as cells in saline alone did not haemolyse, neither was haemolysis eliminated by the use of a different batch of Microtitre plates. It was thought possible that the erythrocytes may have been reacting in some way with the murine sera as it was known that the strain of chicken and preparation of red cells was different at the two centres.

Experiment 3 was carried out to see whether erythrocytes harvested from aged chickens would give comparable results with those used by Heath. Samples of sera were tested in duplicate, one sample with Heath erythrocytes and one sample with CRC erythrocytes. The results showed that identical titres were obtained, the same result being obtained when the experiment was repeated. No work was performed to determine whether receptor sites on the erythrocytes were responsible for the haemolysis but it has been noted whilst this test has been in use, that during overnight adsorption of sera with red cells, some sera haemolyse the cells. It is of interest that this phenomenon has also been observed by other workers using porcine adenovirus (Thompson, 1975).

Following the conclusion of the experiments, an appraisal was made of the results and it was decided that the Heath test would be adopted using erythrocytes from aged chickens.

Haemagglutination Inhibition Test for Pneumonia Virus of Mice

Introduction

When the number of rodents in the barrier unit reached 5000 it was decided to commence screening for the presence of pneumonia virus of mice (PVM). A literature search revealed scanty details of an HI test for this virus (Parker *et al.*, 1965; Blackmore *et al.*, 1972b). In view of the difficulty already experienced with the test for Sendai virus, it was decided that several aspects of a test for PVM should be investigated.

Materials and Methods

The antigen and positive control antiserum were purchased from Microbiological Associates, Bethseda, Maryland, USA. Literature reports (Parker *et al.*, 1965; Blackmore *et al.*, 1972b) stated that mouse erythrocytes should be used in the test. Accordingly these were obtained by exsanguinating aged mice from the barrier maintained breeding unit and collecting the blood in Alsever's solution. After collection the cells were washed three times with phosphate buffered saline and diluted to 0·5%.

The initial test involved the titration of the antigen; doubling dilutions were made using 0·025 ml volumes in a Microtitre plate. Mouse erythrocytes were added and the plate left at room temperature (25°C) for 45 min. After incubation the titration was read and the end point was taken as the dilution showing 50% haemagglutination. The titration was repeated on ten occasions and the titre obtained was taken as 1 HA unit.

The next test involved the titration of the antiserum. Doubling dilutions were made from 1/5 to 1/2560. Antigen diluted to 8 HA units was added to all wells and the plate was left at room temperature for 45 min, after which 0·5% erythrocytes were added and the plate left for a further 30 min. The plate was read and the titre of the serum was taken as the highest dilution showing a complete button of red blood cells. When consistent results were obtained it was considered that the test had been successfully standardized.

An experiment was performed to study the effect of using erythrocytes from various strains of mouse and to see whether chicken red blood cells could be used. Experiment 1 was set up in triplicate using erythrocytes from TO/Crc, NZB/Crc and CBA/H-T6 Crc strain mice. The titres obtained with these cells were identical. In experiment 2 the antigen was titrated with chicken cells and the titre obtained. However, consistent results could not be achieved and it was therefore concluded that the test should be performed with mouse erythrocytes.

Results

It was found that the stated titre of the antigen and antiserum could be repeatedly obtained using the principles of the Heath test. Sera were diluted 1/5 for adsorption and this procedure was carried out at 4°C overnight.

Experiment 1 designed to compare erythrocytes from different strains of mouse yielded comparable results with all sera tested. No correlation was achieved in experiment 2 when chicken erythrocytes were used and therefore all tests were performed using murine erythrocytes.

Discussion

When testing commenced, mouse erythrocytes were obtained from aged TO/Crc mice issued from the barrier unit. Preliminary tests showed that accurate results could be obtained using only 0·025 ml volumes and the quoted titres of both the commercial antigen and antiserum were verified.

Caution was exercised remembering the difficulties experienced with the Sendai test, and pilot tests were performed using murine sera. These were successful but a disturbing feature of each was a degree of haemolysis. It was observed that when mouse red blood cells were kept for longer than 72 h, haemolysis increased rapidly. Therefore, an experiment was performed to examine several strains of mouse as donors of red cells and also whether chicken erythrocytes could be used.

This experiment showed that the strain of mouse cells made no difference to the result and chicken erythrocytes were completely unsuitable as a reagent. As a result of this experiment, murine erythrocytes were used in all subsequent screening.

4

The Microbiological Examination of the Barrier Maintained Breeding Unit

Introduction

Barrier units were introduced into animal houses over 15 years ago to satisfy a demand for an animal of known microbiological status. Prior to their introduction, the status of many of the animals bred for research purposes was dubious and an unknown quantity. It was conceived that by starting with stock free from microorganisms and holding them for subsequent breeding in a barrier unit, the progeny would be of the high status required. As the level of contamination by microorganisms for each animal is known they are termed specified pathogen free (SPF).

The derivation of the initial breeding animals may be by one of two routes, each designed to limit the risk of contamination. For small animals such as rodents, where there is no need to retain the mother, a hysterectomy is performed and the foetuses raised as germ free animals in an isolator from which they are passed into the unit. If larger animals are to be bred, the technique used is a caesarean operation so that the female may be retained for further breeding.

Since the introduction of these units they have become increasingly important in the supply of animals for research, particularly rodents. They permit the breeding and production of animals free from all ecto- and endoparasites and a known list of bacterial and viral agents which may or may not be pathogens. By using animals to this specification, workers at least commence their experiments in the knowledge that complications should not arise due to infections caused by organisms in or on the animals. There have been numerous publications relating to the factors necessary to maintain a barrier unit and Bleby (1976) specified building design and management procedures. Barrier breeding units may be built as a separate building or as an integral part of the animal facility.

At the Clinical Research Centre the barrier unit is built into the Animal House and, when the building was commissioned, it was decided to limit production to rats and mice. It was hoped that in the long term the unit would produce most of the rodents required by workers.

The unit in use utilizes a variety of barriers. They are designed to exclude vermin, microorganisms and to prevent the entry of unauthorized personnel. Efficient ventilation is essential to ensure the exclusion of microorganisms and this is achieved by a combination of air filters (Fig. 5) and the maintenance of positive pressure. The air supply is adjusted so that the air pressure inside the unit is positive to the outside; hence air flow is always from the inside to outside the unit, and this provides the most important barrier. Located in the air supply ducting are filters capable of removing particles to a size of 0·01 μm so that air entering the unit is free from microorganisms. Other barriers used are physical in nature. Staff entering the unit do so through an air lock to a shower after which a completely clean set of clothes is put on. An autoclave (Fig. 6) is provided for the sterilization of all food, bedding, animal boxes and all other non-heat labile materials entering the unit. Any heat labile materials are passed through a disinfectant dunk-tank (Fig. 7) containing 2% Hycolin (William Pearson Ltd, Hull, North Humberside).

The building and equipping of the barrier maintained unit was eventually completed in 1972 and was populated after a strict cleansing and disinfection procedure. After the unit had been cleaned all rooms were sterilized by two fumigations with formalin vapour at an interval of 7 days. The vapour was generated by an electrical element in buckets which were placed at several sites. The air supply system was switched off and the vapour left to fumigate the rooms for 24 h before the air supply was reconnected. Staff entered the unit after showering and a change of clothes, and they fumigated the unit a second time in the same way as the first. Blood agar settle plates were left at several sites as soon as the second fumigation was completed. After 8 h exposure and subsequent incubation at 37°C, none of the plates showed any growth and hence it was felt that the unit was free from bacterial contamination.

The first animals introduced were germ free TO mice which had been reassociated with a mixture of *Escherichia coli, Lactobacillus lactis* and *acidophilus, Bacteroides* species, *Sphaerophorus* species and Enterococcus species. The mice were packed into sterile screw capped jars inside the barrier unit at the National Institute for Medical Research and were then transported to this Centre. On arrival, the jars were passed through

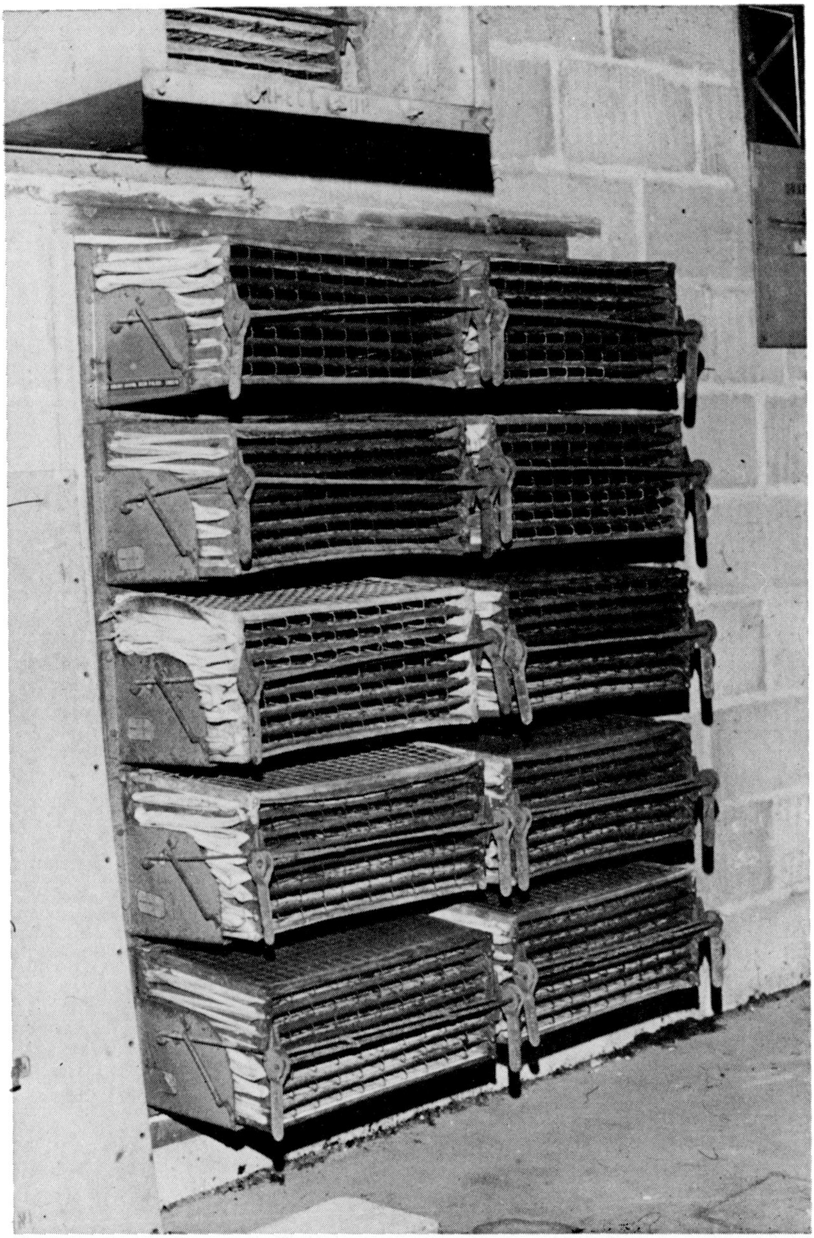

Fig. 5. Barrier unit air inlet primary filters.

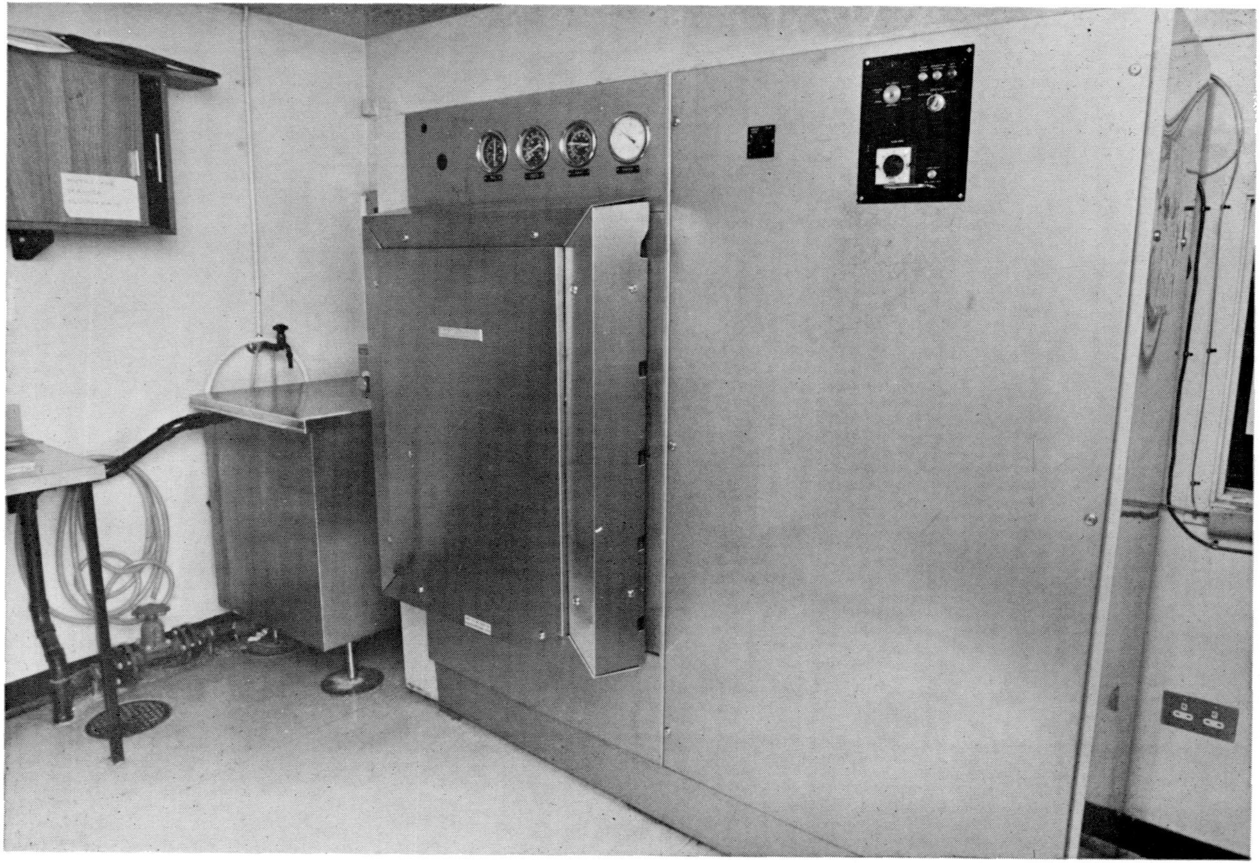

Fig. 6. Barrier unit autoclave and disinfectant dunk tank.

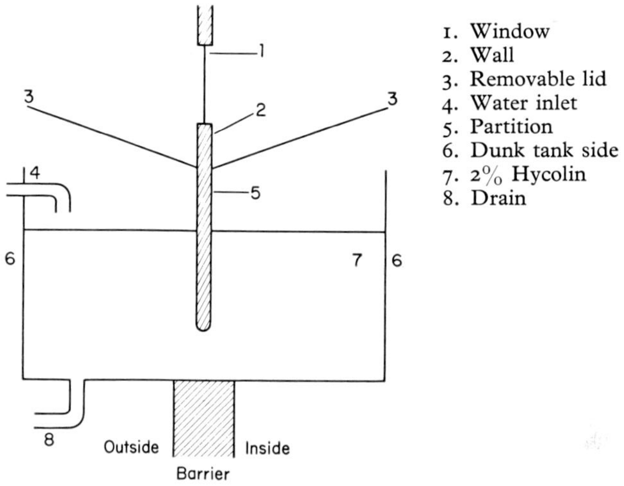

Fig. 7. Sectional view of barrier unit disinfectant dunk tank.

the disinfectant dunk tank and the mice transferred to holding boxes. No health checks were made and the animals were allowed to breed. When the litters were 10 days old a sample was screened as has been described in Chapter 2 (Fig. 1). These checks showed that the animals were only colonized by the organisms in the reassociation mixture. The mice were allowed to continue breeding, so providing the nucleus of stock and also a supply of foster mothers for suckling hysterectomy derived pups from other strains of mice.

These were introduced into the unit over a period of some months (Table 10). The pregnant females were held in conventional rooms near the service area adjacent to the barrier unit. No health checks were made on the donor females. The foetuses were introduced into the unit by hysterectomy, which was performed in the service area under a protective hood in the case of mice, but on the open bench for rats. Normal aseptic precautions were taken; the gravid uterus was passed through the dunk tank in a glass jar containing a weak disinfectant, 10% formalin in 10% tego (Th. Goldschmidt AG, Eastcote, Middx). Inside the unit the foetuses were removed and placed in a box with the young of a female that had littered down 24 h before. The young were left with the foster female for 48 h after which all but two of her own litter were removed and the foster litter left until weaning.

Following the commissioning of a barrier unit there are many points that must be regularly checked to ensure that the unit maintains the quality of animals being issued. It was decided at the outset of the

Table 10

Time of introduction of mice and rats after commissioning of the barrier unit

Species	Strain	Weeks after commissioning	Source
Mouse	TO	4	NIMR
Mouse	CBA/H-T6 Crc	27	CRC
Mouse	C3H-mg/Crc	29	CRC
Mouse	AKR/Crc	29	CRC
Mouse	NUDE	30	CRC
Mouse	BALB/cCrc	31	CRC
Mouse	CBA/CaCrc	32	CRC
Mouse	C57BL/10ScSnCrc	52	CRC
Mouse	A/Crc	52	CRC
Mouse	DBA/2Crc	78	CRC
Rat	SD	57	OLAC
Rat	AGUS/Crc	72	CRC
Rat	PVG/C Crc	73	CRC

NIMR, National Institute for Medical Research; CRC, Clinical Research Centre.

breeding programme that all aspects of the production of animals within the unit were to be studied. These were to include the animals themselves, the staff, the equipment and the environment. A great deal of work was performed involving tests conducted on a quality control basis on the animals issued direct from the unit. These tests were divided into healthy animals examined routinely (572 mice and 92 rats) and those examined because they appeared unwell (93 mice and 35 rats). It is obvious that all apparently sick animals are a hazard to the barrier and must, therefore, be removed speedily and examined. Routine checks on staff were limited to the examination of nasal swabs for the carriage of pathogens. Tests of the autoclave function were carried out weekly and the disinfectant dunk tank was microbiologically tested monthly. Minimal checks were carried out on the environment and these included settle plate analysis of airborne microorganisms and checks on the microbiological content of the water.

Microbiological Screening of Animals

Materials and Methods

A sample of animals was brought out for screening 10 days after the introduction of the first litter of each strain into the unit. When, in turn, these were breeding well and each strain became established, four animals were screened each month. After 1 year, there were approximately 2000 animals inside the unit and the sampling schedule was modified. It was decided that each strain would be examined once every 6 weeks and that a sample size of 18 was to be used. This number was to be made up of three batches of six animals, one batch 3 weeks old, another 9–12 weeks of age and the third taken from ex-breeding pairs. In each age group three male and three female mice were examined and all 18 animals were screened on the same day.

Animals were subjected to the full *post mortem* examination described in Chapter 2 (Fig. 1). Any rodent submitted for examination with clinical signs of illness was subjected to additional tests. Several mice were issued with abscesses on various sites of the body; in all cases pus was removed and culture was attempted using blood agar plates. Other animals appeared to have signs of middle ear disease. Samples were obtained from the middle ear at *post mortem* examination and were cultured on blood agar plates, serum agar and in mycoplasma broth. Animals with suspected respiratory illness were not subjected to additional tests.

Virological testing was confined to serology to detect antibodies against Sendai virus, pneumonia virus of mice (PVM) and animal inoculation for Ectromelia virus. Tests for antibodies against mouse hepatitis virus (MHV), Polyoma virus and Reo III were conducted by a commercial laboratory. Virus tests were carried out using a pool of serum taken from male mice and another from female mice from each age group of animals sampled.

Results

The results of the bacteriological examination of mice are summarized in Tables 11 and 12 and the virological tests in Tables 13 and 14. *Staphylococcus aureus* and *Escherichia coli* were frequently isolated. The latter was found in up to 21% of throat samples and it was noted that the rate of isolation of these two bacteria did not differ significantly when healthy and sick mice were compared. *Staphylococcus aureus* was first isolated 4

Table 11

Percentage isolation of organisms from routine examinations of mice

Mouse strain	Number examined	Organism isolated	Site of isolation and percentage isolation		
			Throat	Lung	Caecum
TO/Crc	178	*Staphylococcus aureus*	64	3	—
		Escherichia coli	7	—	25
		Pseudomonas aeruginosa	—	—	1·5
CBA/H-T6/Crc	48	*Staphylococcus aureus*	65	—	—
		Escherichia coli	—	—	33
C3H-*mg*/Crc	117	*Staphylococcus aureus*	70	2	—
		Escherichia coli	13	—	30
AKR/Crc	69	*Staphylococcus aureus*	23	—	—
		Escherichia coli	7	—	10
BALB/c Crc	20	*Staphylococcus aureus*	25	—	—
		Escherichia coli	—	—	10
CBA/CaCrc	91	*Staphylococcus aureus*	77	—	—
		Escherichia coli	21	—	2
C57BL/10 ScSnCrc	49	*Staphylococcus aureus*	60	—	—
		Escherichia coli	20	—	20

Table 12

Percentage isolation of organisms from clinically sick mice

Mouse strain	Number examined	Organisms isolated	Site of isolation and percentage isolation							
			Throat	Lung	Caecum	Abscess	Liver	Kidney	Spleen	Ears
TO/Crc	90	*Staphylococcus aureus*	44	6	—	10	—	2	2	5
		Escherichia coli	16	2	25	—	—	—	—	—
		Pseudomonas aeruginosa	—	3	10	—	2	2	—	—
		Lactobacillus spp.	NT	NT	—	NT	2	NT	NT	NT
NUDE	3	*Staphylococcus aureus*	100	33	—	66	—	—	—	—
		Escherichia coli	33	—	—	—	—	—	—	—
		Pseudomonas aeruginosa	—	—	33	—	—	—	—	—

NT, not tested.

Table 13

Range of antibody titres obtained from virological tests on healthy mice

Virus	Strain of mice	Number of pools examined	Titres
Sendai	TO/Crc	68	1/8–1/16
	CBA/H-T6 Crc	24	1/8–1/16
	C3H-mg/Crc	48	1/8–1/16
	AKR/Crc	36	1/8–1/16
	NUDE	—	—
	BALB/c Crc	10	1/8
	CBA/Ca Crc	36	1/8–1/16
	C57BL/10 ScSnCrc	13	1/8
Pneumonia	TO/Crc	37	1/5–1/10
	CBA/H-T6Crc	25	1/5
	C3H-mg/Crc	30	1/5–1/10
	AKR/Crc	28	1/5–1/10
	NUDE	—	—
	BALB/c Crc	9	1/5
	CBA/Ca Crc	27	1/5–1/10
	C57BL/10 ScSnCrc	20	1/5–1/10
Hepatitis	TO/Crc	13	1/5–1/10
	CBA/H-T6 Crc	4	1/5–1/10
	C3H-mg/Crc	2	1/5–1/10
	CBA/Ca Crc	2	1/10
	C57BL/10 ScSnCrc	1	1/5
Polyoma	TO/Crc	13	1/5–1/20
	CBA/H-T6 Crc	4	1/5–1/10
	C3H-mg/Crc	2	1/10
	CBA/Ca Crc	2	1/10
	C57BL/10 ScSnCrc	1	1/10
Reo III	TO/Crc	7	1/5–1/10
	CBA/H-T6 Crc	4	1/5–1/10
	C3H-mg/Crc	2	1/5–1/10
	CBA/Ca Crc	2	1/5–1/10
	C57BL/10 ScSnCrc	1	1/5
Ectromelia	TO/Crc	6	Negative

Table 14

Range of antibody titres obtained from virological tests on clinically sick mice

Virus	Strain of mice	Number of pools examined	Titres
Sendai	TO/Crc	48	1/8–1/16
	CBA/H-T6 Crc	1	1/8–1/16
	C3H-mg/Crc	2	1/8
	AKR/Crc	1	1/8
	NUDE	1	1/16
	BALB/c Crc	1	1/8
	CBA/Ca Crc	—	—
	C57BL/10 ScSnCrc	—	—
Pneumonia	TO/Crc	24	1/5–1/10
	CBA/H-T6 Crc	1	1/5
	C3H-mg/Crc	3	1/5–1/10
	AKR/Crc	—	—
	NUDE	3	1/5
	BALB/c Crc	2	1/10
	CBA/Ca Crc	—	—
	C57BL/10 ScSnCrc	1	1/5
Hepatitis	TO/Crc	7	1/5
	CBA/H-T6 Crc	1	1/5
	C3H-mg/Crc	1	1/5
	CBA/CaCrc	—	—
	C57BL/10 ScSnCrc	—	—
Polyoma	TO/Crc	7	1/5–1/10
	CBA/H-T6 Crc	1	1/5
	C3H-mg/Crc	1	1/5
	CBA/Ca Crc	—	—
	C57BL/10 ScSnCrc	—	—
Reo III	TO/Crc	4	1/5
	CBA/H-T6 Crc	1	1/5
	C3H-mg/Crc	1	1/10
	CBA/Ca Crc	—	—
	C57BL/10 ScSnCrc	—	—
Ectromelia	TO/Crc	—	—

Table 15

Percentage isolation of organisms from routine examination of rats

Rat strain	Number examined	Organisms isolated	Site of isolation and percentage isolation		
			Throat	Lung	Caecum
SD/Crc	74	*Staphylococcus aureus*	94	3	—
		Escherichia coli	32	—	30
		Pseudomonas aeruginosa	—	—	13
AGUS/Crc	3	*Staphylococcus aureus*	100	100	—
		Escherichia coli	100	—	67
		Pseudomonas aeruginosa	33	—	33
PVG/cCrc	15	*Staphylococcus aureus*	100	—	—
		Escherichia coli	33	—	33

Table 16

Percentage isolation of organisms from clinically sick rats

Rat strain	Number examined	Organism isolated	Site of isolation and percentage isolation				
			Throat	Lung	Caecum	Abscess	Ear
SD/Crc	35	*Staphylococcus aureus*	100	25	—	3	10
		Escherichia coli	50	10	72	—	—

months after the commissioning of the unit. *Pseudomonas aeruginosa* was first isolated after 16 months and was regarded as a contaminant, but was not associated with overt disease outbreaks. Throughout the entire screening programme no evidence of virus infections in mice was detected. Similarly, no mycoplasmas were isolated and nor were endo- or ectoparasites.

The rats examined, whether healthy or sick, were colonized by the same organisms as found in mice (Tables 15 and 16). However, the percentage isolation of these organisms was higher than mice. Serum from each rat was tested for the presence of antibodies to Sendai virus. The titres obtained were within the range of $\frac{1}{8}$–$\frac{1}{16}$. No evidence of endo- or ectoparasites was detected nor were any mycoplasmas isolated.

Microbiological Screening of the Environment

Materials and Methods

Staff Monitoring

Monthly nasal swabs were taken from all staff working within the unit. New or temporary staff were swabbed 4 days prior to entry and where practicable, maintenance staff were swabbed immediately prior to entry into the unit. The swabs were plated on to blood agar and chocolate agar plates and incubated aerobically for 18 h at 37°C. After identification, isolates of *Staphylococcus aureus* were sent for phage typing to the Central Public Health Laboratories, Colindale.

Autoclave and Dunk Tank

The autoclave serving the unit is a Drayton Castle high vacuum machine. It is automatically controlled and a pressure recording chart and temperature recording chart are fitted. A microbiological test of the autoclave function was carried out each week. Two spore strips (Oxoid Ltd, Basingstoke, Hants), impregnated with spores of *Bacillus stearothermophilus,* were placed at the centre of a bag of diet. The autoclave was then loaded and this bag was placed at the centre of the load. After the process was completed the strips were recovered and sent to the laboratory for culture at 56°C in tryptone soya broth for 7 days.

The dunk tank filled with 2% Hycolin is situated adjacent to the autoclave (Fig. 6). Samples of fluid were cultured monthly. A 20 ml sample of fluid was pipetted aseptically into a sterile bottle. 0·1 ml of fluid was spread on two blood agar plates, one incubated aerobically at 37°C and the other anaerobically. 0·1 ml aliquots of fluid were inoculated into four glucose broths and four Robertson's cooked meat medium; two of each medium were incubated at room temperature (25°C) and two at 37°C. Finally the fluid was centrifuged and any deposit present was cultured on blood agar plates.

Water Testing

Testing of the water supply was first instigated after discoloured water was seen on two separate occasions. Samples of water were collected in 500 ml bottles containing a trace of sodium thiosulphate. The tap water samples were treated as described by Baker (1969). Additionally 0·1 ml of each sample was spread on to a blood agar plate for aerobic incubation at 37°C. Following the isolation of *Pseudomonas aeruginosa* from mice issued from the unit, all taps and sinks were examined. Water samples were obtained from 11 sites (Table 17) and swabs were taken from all sink waste pipes. Care was taken to ensure that the walls of the pipe were adequately sampled and no contact was made with the water in the trap. The water samples were treated as before; each swab was inoculated on to two blood agar plates, one plate was incubated at 37°C, the other at room temperature. After incubation all colonies present were identified using normal methods.

Results

Staff Monitoring

All staff working within the unit were found to be persistent carriers of *Staphylococcus aureus*. The organisms were subjected to phage typing but at no time were any of these strains isolated from rodents.

Autoclave and Dunk Tank

On two separate occasions a positive culture was obtained from one of the two spore strips used in the autoclave test, indicating a faulty sterilization procedure. A subsequent retest was satisfactory in each case. At no time were any organisms cultured from samples of dunk tank fluid.

Table 17

Site and result of water sampling

Site	Presumptive coliform count (MacConkey broth)	Plate count 37°C	Plate count 22°C	Swabs: Organism isolated
Rodent rooms				
3Y031	Nil	Nil	Nil	*P. fluorescens*
3Y030	Nil	Nil	Nil	*P. fluorescens*
3Y029	Nil	2 colonies/ml	150 colonies/ml	*P. fluorescens*
3Y028	Nil	Nil	Nil	*P. fluorescens*
3Y027	Nil	Nil	130 colonies/ml	*P. fluorescens*
Female toilet sink	Nil	Nil	Nil	*P. fluorescens*
Male toilet sink	Nil	Nil	60 colonies/ml	*P. fluorescens*
Common room	Nil	Nil	Nil	No isolates
Laundry sink	Nil	Nil	Nil	*P. fluorescens*
Cage washing tank tap 1	Nil	Nil	Nil	No isolates
Cage washing tank tap 2	Nil	Nil	Nil	No isolates

Water Testing

No organisms were isolated on either occasion when discoloured water was noticed and tested. Moreover, only one organism was isolated when all taps and sinks were tested. *Pseudomonas fluorescens* was present in the sinks of all animal holding rooms although not in the cage washing tanks (Table 17). The presumptive coliform count in all tests was negative. Water samples from three rooms yielded small numbers of organisms when incubated at 22°C, but none when incubation was performed at 37°C. This indicated that the organisms were saprophytes and therefore not potential pathogens.

Discussion

A barrier unit's objective is to provide the research worker with an animal, free from microorganisms that will adversely affect his experimental results. These animals are generally termed Specific Pathogen Free animals. The policy from the commencement of breeding in the unit was to exclude as many organisms as possible. The original mice were reassociated with a mixture of *Escherichia coli, Lactobacillus lactis* and *acidophilus, Bacteroides* species, *Sphaerophorus* species and Enterococcus species and it was hoped that it would be possible to keep the rodents free from all other organisms. This was not to be the case. *Staphylococcus aureus* was found to be a contaminant organism 4 months after the unit was commissioned. The organism was responsible for overt disease unlike the other contaminant organism, *Pseudomonas aeruginosa,* first isolated 16 months after the unit opened. The studies undertaken to trace the source of these organisms will be discussed below.

The microbiological control of such a production unit is a complex operation and one that commences before the unit is commissioned. It is probably of value to consider the results obtained from the control programme in chronological order.

The unit was sterilized by two formalin fumigations, the first of which revealed many minor structural cracks around door frames, dunk tank and autoclave, due to plaster shrinkage. These were filled before the second fumigation after which blood agar plates left exposed in the unit showed the absence of bacterial contamination. Taylor (1974) reported that fumigation was not sufficient to eliminate organisms. He showed that 13 sites out of 100 tested were contaminated with bacteria after fumigation. He used swabs to collect specimens which gave a very accurate sampling of each site. However, a swab will only collect contamination over a small area whereas settle plates provide a sample of a large area. This is a great advantage as they provide an "in-use" test of each area over a long period of time (8 h), testing the air filtration system and dissemination of organisms by staff and apparatus.

The various strains of rodents were introduced into the unit over a period of 78 weeks after commissioning (Table 10). The original TO mice were introduced from the National Institute for Medical Research, Mill Hill. These bred successfully and formed the nucleus of foster mothers. Other strains were introduced from the conventional breeding colony by hysterectomy technique. No health checks were performed on the donor animals. This could have exposed the unit to bacterial contamination as Casillo and Blackmore (1972) published the results of a survey, showing that 8·2% of the uteri from animals within a conventional colony were infected with *Pasteurella pneumotropica*. If this applies to all conventional mouse colonies it was perhaps fortunate that *Pasteurella pneumotropica* was not introduced into the unit when hysterectomies were performed, as this organism was known to be present in throat samples in all conventional rooms at this Centre. Consideration was given, in the light of this report, to a method of bacteriologically examining the lumen of the gravid uterus but it was felt that the risk to the live foetuses and possible risk of introducing contamination was too great.

Once the numbers of mice bred increased, consideration was given to a realistic sampling schedule. Initially all new litters were examined when 10 days old by the standard protocol already described (Fig. 1). The examination was not as thorough as that recommended by Hill (1966); fewer sites on the animal were examined but it was felt that this was counter balanced by sampling more animals at shorter intervals. The screening of the animals, some 792 in all, revealed consistent results that are displayed in Tables 11–14. Only two contaminant organisms were isolated which compares favourably with experience at other centres; for example Walburg *et al.* (1965) reported contamination by five genera of bacteria. *Escherichia coli,* which was one of the bacteria used in the deliberate reassociation of gut flora, was frequently isolated together with the contaminant *Staphylococcus aureus.* This latter organism was first isolated 4 months after the unit began production. It was soon apparent that the organism was the cause of clinical lesions in some animals. These lesions were normally seen as mammary abscesses, bulbourethral gland infections (Needham and Cooper, 1976) which resemble those described by Sebesteny (1973) caused by *Pasteurella pneumotropica,* and also as abscesses on various other areas of the body resulting from fight wounds. The presence of these various lesions necessitated rigorous culling as affected animals were obviously totally unsuitable for issue.

Several investigations were undertaken to try and trace the source of the *Staphylococcus aureus.* Isolates of the organism from the rodents and all staff involved with the unit were sent to the Central Public Health Laboratory, Colindale, for phage typing. This showed that several phage types of *Staphylococcus aureus* were present in the animals as shown in Table 18. A small percentage (0·1%) of strains were untypable, which contrasted with the experience of other workers; Morrison *et al.* (1961) found 102 out of 123 isolates from dogs, cats, cattle and horses were untypable when using human phage types, whilst Mann and Bjotvedt (1966) found 89% of staphylococci from 12 species of animals were untypable. The high proportion of human phage types isolated from the animals within the unit suggested that the introduction of this organism was by human transmission to the animals, although in fact the isolates of staphylococci obtained from the staff regularly employed in the unit and the animals were not the same. This differed to a similar outbreak

Table 18

Phage types and percentage isolation of *Staphylococcus aureus* in mice

Phage type of *Staphylococcus aureus*	% isolation
6. 47. 53. 54. 75. 85.	42·0
29. 52. 6. 47. 53. 54. 75. 85.	7·0
6. 47. 53. 54. 75. 84. 85.	21·0
6. 47. 54. 75. 85.	2·0
29. 52. 80. 6. 47. 53. 54. 75. 83A. 85.	12·0
6. 53. 54. 75. 85.	14·0
6. 54. 75. 83A. 85.	2·0

described by Blackmore and Francis (1970) who were able to demonstrate the isolation of similar phage types from the animals and staff involved. On this evidence, further consideration was given to the possible routes by which this organism could have entered. The filters in the air supply ducting could have been at fault but in this case other organisms would have been detected. During the period immediately prior to the appearance of the staphylococcus, it was known that due to an electrical fault the supply fans stopped and then ran in reverse; the resultant negative pressure would have drawn air into the unit, so bypassing the air filtration unit. However, it was felt that this was unlikely to be the cause of bacterial contamination as again other organisms would have been drawn in. The route of entry of the *Staphylococcus aureus* was never established. Recently, Clark *et al.* (1978) reported that the source of contamination by *Staphylococcus aureus* within their unit could not be traced.

The findings at this Centre, together with their's suggests that it is probably impossible to trace the source of such a ubiquitous bacterium. That the animals were colonized by this organism had to be accepted as irrevocable and the only way of eradication would have been the drastic and impracticable step of culling affected stock and building up the colony again. Treatment of all animals was considered as an alternative method of eradication. However, it was decided that as the supply of rodents from the unit was not severely disrupted and it was found by experiment (see Experimental Investigations, Chapter 6) that the organism was replaced by commensal bacteria when the mice were issued to conventional rooms, treatment with antibiotics or by immunization (Hill, 1969) would be counterproductive.

Regular testing showed that the various strains of mice were colonized by *Staphylococcus aureus* to different degrees (Table 11). Within one room, for example, 77% of the throats of CBA/CaCrc mice were colonized with the organism compared with only 23% of AKR/Crc strain throat samples. A possible explanation for this observation is that some strains of mice are more able to naturally resist infection by this organism than others.

The appearance of *Pseudomonas aeruginosa* in mice 16 months after the start of the breeding programmes prompted a full scale water test. It was known that the water piped to the unit was unsterilized and was fed directly from pressure tanks situated in the Hospital. The test showed that *Pseudomonas fluorescens* was present in the sink traps of all the animal rooms but that overall the standard of the water supplied was good. In all water tests the presumptive coliform count was nil and the saprophyte count was entirely satisfactory in the absence of potential pathogens. Once again the source of a contaminant organism was not traced although it was thought to be water borne. However, the number of animals colonized by this organism was very small and hence no steps were introduced to sterilize the water supply.

The other area checked frequently as a source of possible contamination was the service area autoclave and dunk tank. On two occasions the autoclave gave unsatisfactory results. Each time one of the two spore strips in the test was not sterilized. As only one strip was involved interpretation of the test was difficult as in the case of a failure to sterilize it would be expected that both strips would grow. No reasonable explanation for this phenomenon could be found, but an immediate retest of the autoclave, without any adjustments being made to the cycling procedure, yielded satisfactory results.

The screening programme has proved essential to the efficient management of the barrier unit and without the tests the unit's function would have been impaired. By definition the animals issued are free from specified pathogens and hence the constant microbiological evaluation of the animals allows the species of organisms present to be known. The tests have shown that apart from two contaminant organisms the animals are still only colonized by the bacteria contained in the reassociation mixture. The subsequent issue of these high quality animals has meant that experiments have proceeded without disease problems and that the level of microorganisms within the Animal House has remained low.

In addition to screening animals, the programme has also proved of great value in the maintenance of a defined environment in the unit by testing autoclave function, water supplies and possible contamination by staff. Without all these tests the whole concept of a barrier unit could not be maintained.

5

The Microbiological Screening of Conventionally Housed Mice

Animals and Equipment

Introduction

Conventionally housed mice form the largest group of animals within the facility. They are kept in polypropylene boxes on wood chip bedding in eight rooms. There are no barriers involved and all rooms are fully accessible to research workers. The rooms are situated on two floors of the building; the upper floor (level 3) originally housed the breeding colony but now houses animals of barrier unit origin or animals of category **** status (Laboratory Animals Centre (LAC) accreditation scheme, Townsend, 1969) whereas the lower floor (level 2) houses all rodents that are not derived from the afore-mentioned categories (see Appendices 2 and 3). Included among the animals are many mice that are involved in long term immunological experiments and may have undergone such procedures as splenectomy, adrenalectomy, X-ray irradiation, immunosuppressant therapy and thymectomy, each designed to modify the immune response of the animals concerned.

The quality control screening of conventional mice was organized in five categories:

(1) Routine sampling of mice bred by conventional mating in the breeding colony prior to the commissioning of the barrier maintained unit.

(2) The examination of clinically sick mice from the breeding colony.

(3) Sampling at set intervals of mice which were held in conven-

tional rooms to monitor build up of microorganisms (designated sentinel mice).

(4) Examination of mice at the request of research workers.

(5) Examination of mice from laboratory animal breeders.

Breeding Colony

The breeding colony was established in three rooms, with outbred TO strain mice in one and various inbred strains in the other two. The mice forming this colony were used as the source of pregnant females to provide litters for introduction into the barrier unit. When this was commissioned, two of the rooms were redesignated for holding rodents in experiments and one remained as a breeding room for special projects. Each strain of mouse was examined microbiologically once a month. Normally, four 3-week-old mice or four ex-breeders were screened. The frequency of sampling was gradually reduced as production of rodents increased in the barrier unit.

Sick Mice from the Breeding Colony

Any mice in the breeding unit appearing clinically sick were subjected to the full screening protocol (Fig. 1) (see Chapter 2). It was usual for all the mice in the box to be examined irrespective of how many animals within that box were showing symptoms of disease. The most frequently observed condition was diarrhoea, whilst respiratory conditions occurred infrequently.

Sentinel Mice

It had been decided that the microbiological status of all rooms housing rodents, including the infected suite, should be monitored continually. This was achieved by the use of sentinel mice. These were male TO/Crc strain, 4 weeks old, issued from the barrier maintained breeding unit. Immediately on issue, four mice were fully examined as previously described, in order that base line data could be obtained. They were then placed 10 to a box, two boxes to a room, where they remained for up to 6 months. One box was placed near the air supply inlet, the other near the extract. In the infected suite one box was placed in the lobby, one in the service area and one in the room holding the isolators. Once in position, the boxes were not moved and were managed under normal husbandry methods. Two mice were examined from each box once a month.

Research Workers Requests

With as many as 20 000 experimental mice on site at any one time, it was realized that research workers might easily encounter unexpected clinical illness amongst their animals. In the event, requests were received from many workers to examine not only animals which were obviously sick, but those from which aberrant experimental results had been obtained.

Laboratory Mice Suppliers

As it was known that large numbers of mice would have to be bought from commercial sources, until the barrier unit was producing sufficient animals, it was thought essential to examine animals from commercial breeders. Immediately on arrival at this Centre a sample of animals was microbiologically examined.

It was also decided that checks should be carried out on the environment of the Animal House. Apart from the rooms which were to be monitored by sentinel mice it was decided to examine the autoclave and disinfectant footpads in the infected suite, as well as the cage wash machine, on a regular basis.

During the course of the routine investigations just outlined, it became apparent from the results obtained in certain areas of the work that further investigation was warranted. This involved investigating in depth the colonization of mouse throats by bacteria, liver infections in apparently healthy mice and the difference in infection rates between male and female mice. The three experiments are recorded in Chapter 6.

Materials and Methods

Animals

Each strain of mouse in the breeding colony was sampled approximately once a month, sampling four mice at a time. Sick animals were examined when necessary and the numbers and ages varied, the youngest being 10 days old.

Sentinel mice were examined at approximately monthly intervals, two mice being taken from each box.

Mice examined at the request of research workers varied in numbers and mice of many strains and both sexes were involved. In some cases experimental work had not started but animals were screened at the request of the worker prior to use, because results of a previous experiment had appeared to be dubious.

Mice from commercial suppliers were examined in one of two ways. If a single batch was delivered, a random sample of up to ten animals was

Table 19

Number of conventional mice examined and location

Source and room number	Reason for sample	Number of batches examined	Total number of mice examined
Infected suite	Sentinels	30	106
2Y039	Sentinels	13	57
2Y040	Sentinels	25	105
2Y041	Sentinels	20	75
2Y042	Sentinels	19	77
2Y043	Sentinels	25	106
3Y033	Sentinels	8	31
3Y034	Sentinels	17	67
3Y035	Sentinels	7	28
3Y036	Sentinels	5	20
3Y037	Sentinels	13	57
Outside suppliers	Quality control	39	222
3Y034	Breeding colony routine	25	111
3Y034	Breeding colony queries	22	57
3Y035	Breeding colony routine	35	148
3Y035	Breeding colony queries	28	104
3Y037	Breeding colony routine	6	40
3Y037	Breeding colony queries	5	30
All holding rooms	Research workers queries	109	528

taken; however where a standing order had been placed with a commercial source, three mice of each sex were examined for five consecutive deliveries.

The total numbers of mice from the above categories submitted for examination are shown in Table 19.

Methods

Each animal was subjected to the full screening protocol already described (Fig. 1). Variations to this protocol were made where necessary.

In cases of severe diarrhoea involving mice from the breeding colony, blood was obtained and only caecal contents were examined bacteriologically. Sentinel mice were carefully examined and it was found that in several cases liver lesions were present. The detailed investigation of this condition will be reported in Chapter 6.

Mice involved in experiments were subjected to careful scrutiny and specimens taken according to the suspected illness. Lymph nodes of immunosuppressed animals were examined and if thought to be enlarged, were placed in 10% formal saline prior to histological examination.

Serum taken from all mice examined was tested for the presence of antibodies to Sendai virus. No other virological tests were carried out on any of the mice, except the sentinel mice. Pools of serum from these animals were examined for the presence of antibodies to Polyoma, Reo III and mouse hepatitis virus. One pool of serum from each room was tested at the end of the first 6 months after quality control screening had been instituted. Six months later another pool of serum was tested followed by another after 2 months and another after a further 2 months. This provided information on the virological status of each room over an 18 month period since when testing has continued on a 6 monthly schedule.

The infected suite autoclave was tested 128 times. On each occasion two spore strips, impregnated with *Bacillus stearothermophilus* spores, were placed at the centre of the load. At the end of the cycle these were recovered and cultured in tryptone soya broth at 56°C for 7 days. The disinfectant footpads in the suite were tested less frequently. These consisted of a rectangular depression in the floor, filled with a piece of foam rubber which was soaked in 5% chloros (ICI, Durham Chemical Distributors Ltd, Birtley, Co. Durham). When tests were carried out, a blood agar plate was gently pressed on to the driest part of the mat and subsequently cultured at 37°C for 48 h.

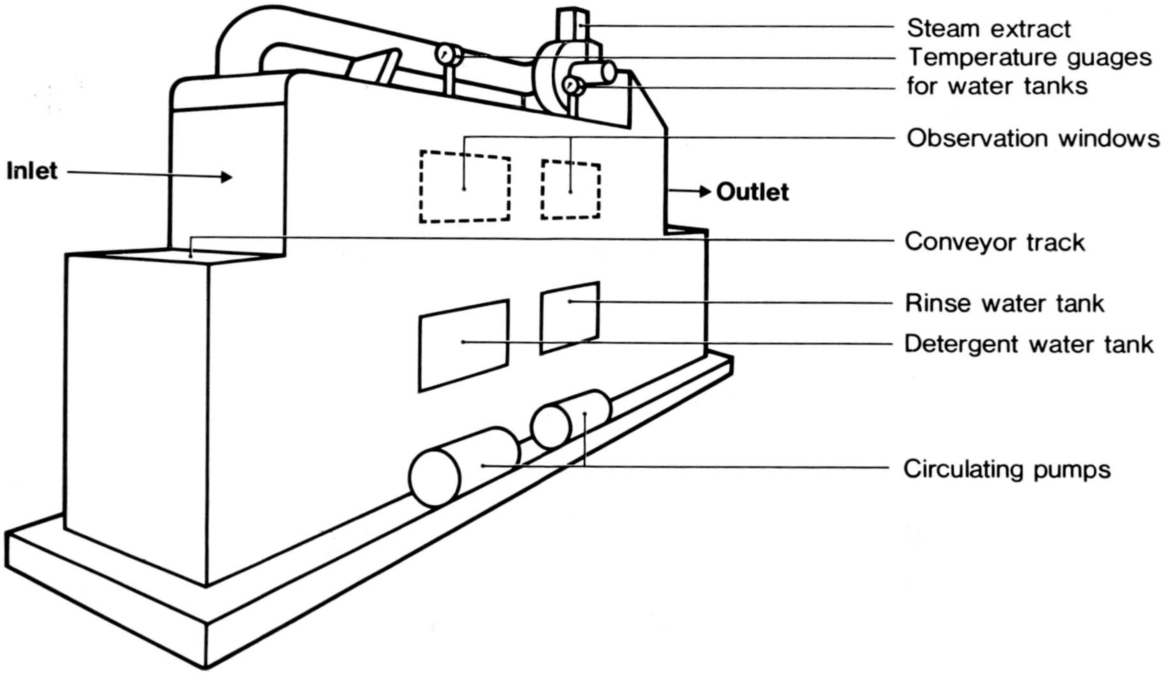

Fig. 8. Conveyor tunnel cage wash machine.

Dirty cages are subjected to a three cycle cleansing process in a tunnel washer equipped with a detergent tank, a rinse tank and a steam sterilizer (Fig. 8). It was decided to monitor the efficiency of the washer, check the washed boxes for sterility and to determine the microbiological status of each water tank. Samples of the detergent tank water were withdrawn at the start of the process and then half-hourly until the end of the wash. On every occasion that the tank was sampled the temperature of the water was recorded. This was repeated for the rinse tank. In the laboratory, 0·1 ml of each sample was spread on to a blood agar plate which was incubated at 37°C for 18 h. At each sample time the inside of a freshly washed box was swabbed and the swab was plated on to a blood agar plate which was incubated at 37°C for 18 h. After incubation the colonies present were counted and identified according to Cowan and Steel (1966). Samples were taken each day for 4 weeks.

Results

Breeding Colony

The mice in the breeding colony were screened either as routine samples at set intervals or examined when clinically ill (Table 20). It was found that throat samples taken from mice housed in all three rooms yielded *Pasteurella pneumotropica*, *Streptococcus* species and *Proteus* species. In addition, the throats of clinically sick mice were colonized by *Escherichia coli* and *Klebsiella* species. *Pasteurella pneumotropica* was isolated from the lungs of mice in all rooms and lung samples obtained from sick mice also yielded *Proteus* species, *Klebsiella* species and *Streptococcus* species. Mycoplasma was only isolated from the respiratory tracts of inbred strains of mice which were held in two rooms. Samples of faeces from both categories of mice yielded *Proteus* species, *Escherichia coli* and the nematode parasite *Syphacia obvelata*. Caecal contents from sick mice also yielded *Pseudomonas* species and *Klebsiella* species. The ectoparasite *Myobia musculi* was found only on sick inbred mice from one room. All pools of serum tested showed that Sendai virus was present in every room with antibody titres up to $\frac{1}{256}$ being obtained.

Sentinel Mice

Mice from every room showed that *Pasteurella pneumotropica* and *Streptococcus* species frequently colonized the throats. With the excep-

Table 20

Percentage isolation of organisms and range of antibody titres to Sendai virus from mice in the conventional breeding colony

Source	Reason for sample	Percentage isolation: Throat						Lung					Lung and throat	Caecum					Skin	Sendai titre
		E. coli	*P. pneumotropica*	*P. haemolytica*	*Streptococcus* spp.	*Proteus* spp.	*Klebsiella* spp.	*Proteus* spp.	*P. pneumotropica*	*Klebsiella* spp.	*Streptococcus* spp.	*E. coli*	*Mycoplasma* sp.	*Pseudomonas* spp.	*Proteus* spp.	*E. coli*	*Klebsiella* spp.	*S. obvelata*	*M. musculi*	
3Y034	Routine	—	85	—	54	18	—	3	4	—	—	—	7	—	27	7	—	9	—	$\frac{1}{8}-\frac{1}{256}$
3Y035	Routine	—	66	4	58	20	—	—	8	—	—	2	1	—	16	—	—	14	—	$\frac{1}{8}-\frac{1}{64}$
3Y037	Routine	—	70	10	10	8	—	—	10	—	—	1	—	—	20	10	—	30	—	$\frac{1}{8}-\frac{1}{256}$
3Y034	"Sick"	12	46	2	52	28	2	8	8	2	4	—	12	2	12	18	2	8	6	$\frac{1}{8}-\frac{1}{258}$
3Y035	"Sick"	5	31	—	26	10	3	2	5	1	2	2	1	1	10	4	4	3	—	$\frac{1}{10}-\frac{1}{256}$
3Y037	"Sick"	—	13	3	7	60	—	10	30	3	—	—	—	—	7	—	10	7	—	$\frac{1}{16}-\frac{1}{32}$

—, no isolates.

Table 21

Percentage isolation of organisms from sentinel mice

Source	Percentage isolation																
	Throat						Lung			Lung and throat	Caecum					Skin
	P. pneumotropica	*P. haemolytica*	*Streptococcus* spp.	*Klebsiella* spp.	*Proteus* spp.	*E. coli*	*Klebsiella* spp.	*P. pneumotropica*	*Streptococcus* spp.	*Mycoplasma* sp.	*Proteus* spp.	*E. coli*	*Klebsiella* spp.	*Pseudomonas* spp.	*S. obvelata*	*M. musculi*
Infected suite	8	—	59	—	—	7	—	—	—	—	—	4	—	5	—	—
2Y039	62	—	74	12	8	—	—	8	2	—	16	4	—	—	38	6
2Y040	63	5	75	8	2	1	1	1	—	6	11	4	1	—	12	4
2Y041	44	3	80	—	5	1	—	1	—	8	3	12	—	—	1	—
2Y042	60	—	76	—	—	—	—	3	1	4	—	3	—	—	1	—
2Y043	68	5	89	6	3	—	—	1	—	3	10	—	2	—	26	10
3Y033	72	—	62	—	—	—	—	3	—	4	2	2	2	—	—	—
3Y034	55	—	52	—	—	—	10	5	4	—	—	5	—	—	—	—
3Y035	54	—	33	—	—	—	4	8	—	—	4	—	13	—	7	—
3Y036	51	—	71	—	—	—	—	4	3	6	—	5	—	—	4	—
3Y037	66	—	72	—	—	—	—	9	9	—	—	9	—	—	12	—

—, no isolates

tion of samples taken from mice in the infected suite, *Pasteurella pneumotropica* was isolated from up to 9% of lungs. Sentinel mice first became infected with *Mycoplasma* species 4 weeks after being placed in a holding room and as can be seen in Table 21, six of the 11 areas monitored were affected by this species of organism. Within a similar period of time *Proteus* species was first isolated from throat samples obtained from mice in four rooms. Serological tests for the presence of antibodies to Sendai virus performed on pools of serum obtained from each batch of mice examined, demonstrated that this virus was present in every room and antibody titres of $\frac{1}{256}$ were obtained. No evidence of antibodies to mouse hepatitis virus or Reo III was found although one room was found to be infected with Polyoma virus (Table 22). The endoparasite *Syphacia obvelata* was found in the faeces of mice from eight rooms, and the ectoparasite *Myobia musculi* was seen on mice from only three rooms.

Table 22

Range of antibody titres to murine viruses from sentinel mice

	Range of virus titres			
Source	Sendai	Reo III	Hepatitis	Polyoma
Infected suite	$\frac{1}{8}$–$\frac{1}{128}$	$\frac{1}{5}$	$\frac{1}{5}$–$\frac{1}{20}$	$\frac{1}{5}$
2Y039	$\frac{1}{8}$–$\frac{1}{128}$	–	–	–
2Y040	$\frac{1}{8}$–$\frac{1}{128}$	$\frac{1}{5}$	$\frac{1}{5}$	$\frac{1}{5}$
2Y041	$\frac{1}{8}$–$\frac{1}{256}$	$\frac{1}{5}$	$\frac{1}{5}$	$\frac{1}{5}$
2Y042	$\frac{1}{12}$–$\frac{1}{256}$	$\frac{1}{5}$	$\frac{1}{5}$	$\frac{1}{5}$
2Y043	$\frac{1}{8}$–$\frac{1}{256}$	$\frac{1}{5}$–$\frac{1}{20}$	$\frac{1}{5}$	$\frac{1}{5}$–$\frac{1}{20}$
3Y033	$\frac{1}{8}$–$\frac{1}{256}$	$\frac{1}{5}$–$\frac{1}{10}$	$\frac{1}{5}$	$\frac{1}{40}$–$\frac{1}{160}$
3Y034	$\frac{1}{8}$–$\frac{1}{128}$	$\frac{1}{5}$	$\frac{1}{5}$	$\frac{1}{5}$–$\frac{1}{20}$
3Y035	$\frac{1}{8}$–$\frac{1}{128}$	$\frac{1}{5}$–$\frac{1}{10}$	$\frac{1}{5}$–$\frac{1}{10}$	$\frac{1}{5}$–$\frac{1}{40}$
3Y036	$\frac{1}{8}$–$\frac{1}{128}$	$\frac{1}{5}$–$\frac{1}{10}$	$\frac{1}{5}$	$\frac{1}{5}$–$\frac{1}{20}$
3Y037	$\frac{1}{8}$–$\frac{1}{128}$	$\frac{1}{5}$–$\frac{1}{10}$	$\frac{1}{5}$	$\frac{1}{5}$–$\frac{1}{10}$

Clinically Sick Experimental Mice

Throat, lung and faecal samples from experimental mice that were clinically sick yielded a similar spectrum of organisms encountered in all

Table 23

Percentage isolation of organisms and range of antibody titres to Sendai virus from research workers "sick" mice

Percentage isolation																	
Throat					Lung			Lung and throat	Caecum					Skin		Sendai titre
E. coli	*Proteus* spp.	*P. haemolytica*	*Streptococcus* spp.	*P. pneumotropica*	*E. coli*	*P. pneumotropica*	*Proteus* spp.	*Mycoplasma* sp.	*Klebsiella* spp.	*E. coli*	*Proteus* spp.	*S. obvelata*	*H. nana*	*M. musculinus*	*M. musculi*	
4	8	3	34	30	2	10	2	7	1	6	10	8	2	3	13	$\frac{1}{8}$–$\frac{1}{512}$

Table 24

Percentage isolation of organisms and range of antibody titres to Sendai virus from mice obtained from commercial sources

Percentage Isolation															
Throat				Lung				Lung and throat	Caecum			Skin		Sendai titre
E. coli	*Proteus* spp.	*P. pneumotropica*	*Enterobacter* spp.	*Streptococcus* spp.	*P. pneumotropica*	*Proteus* sp.	*Enterobacter* spp.	*Mycoplasma* sp.	*Proteus* spp.	*E. coli*	*S. obvelata*	*M. musculinus*	*M. musculi*	
11	30	12	6	26	2·5	5	2·5	1·5[a]	15	5	3[b]	0·5[c]	0·5[c]	$\frac{1}{8}$–$\frac{1}{256}$

[a] found in mice from supplier A only.
[b] found in mice from supplier B only.
[c] found in mice from supplier C only.

the other categories of mice (Table 23). Additionally the endoparasite *Hymenolepis nana* was found in 2% of faecal samples. Three percent of mice were infested with *Myocoptes musculinus* and 13% with *Myobia musculi*. Pools of serum tested for antibodies to Sendai virus showed evidence of infection and titres of $\frac{1}{512}$ were obtained.

Mice from Commercial Sources

A high proportion (30%) of the throats of mice delivered to this Centre were colonized with *Proteus* species (Table 24). Three suppliers delivered batches of mice colonized with microorganisms considered to be undesirable. Mice from supplier A were colonized with a *Mycoplasma* species, supplier B delivered mice infested with the ectoparasites *Myocoptes musculinus* and *Myobia musculi* and animals from supplier C were colonized with *Syphacia obvelata*. Pools of serum from mice supplied from several commercial breeders were found to have significant Sendai antibody titres.

The autoclave function tests showed that the sterilizing cycle in operation was entirely satisfactory. The blood agar plate used to sample the disinfectant footpads in the infected suite usually yielded less than ten colonies identified as *Bacillus* species. The preliminary experiments with the cage washer showed that all boxes examined contained bacteria which were identified as *Bacillus* species in the majority of cases, although on isolated occasions *Staphylococcus aureus* and *Escherichia coli* were recovered. Large numbers of organisms, often in excess of 3000/ml were isolated from the detergent tank but lower numbers of organisms were recovered from the rinse tank. The temperatures of both tanks varied greatly during the wash cycle with temperatures of between 50°C and 100°C being recorded.

Discussion

Several conclusions may be drawn from the screening of the various categories of conventional mice of which a total of 1970 animals were examined.

Within the three rooms comprising the breeding colony, up to 85% of healthy mouse throats were colonized with *Pasteurella pneumotropica*. Between the rooms there was a difference in isolation rates of this organism of 20% (66% to 85%). *Streptococcus* species was isolated from throat samples at approximately equal rates in two rooms (54% in one and 58% in the other) whereas less isolates (10%) were obtained from a third room. This latter room contained outbred TO strain mice and it was found that these were always heavily colonized by *Pasteurella pneumotropica,* which then appeared to suppress the colonization of throats by *Streptococcus* species. Recovery of bacteria from lung samples was never greater than 2% and hence in most mice the lungs were regarded as sterile. Mycoplasmas were occasionally isolated but in only one room were they found consistently. The caeca of the animals yielded only small numbers of normal commensal organisms and pathogens were never isolated. It is likely that the number of commensals detected in this category of mice as in all others was reduced due to the selectivity of the media in use (deoxycholate citrate agar and selenite F). Only one species of parasite was found and this was the endoparasite *Syphacia obvelata*. This nematode worm was found in the caeca of mice from all rooms and in some cases the caecum was half filled with clusters of entwined worms.

Comparison of the results obtained from sick and healthy mice from the breeding colony did not reveal significant differences. In general, sick mice carried a greater number of bacterial species and there was an increased isolation of *Mycoplasma* species. One organism in particular, *Proteus* species, was frequently isolated from the throats of sick mice (in one room up to 60%). Respiratory disease was encountered and more species of bacteria were isolated from lung samples. Much has been written on the aetiology and causal organisms (Bell and Elmes, 1969; Brennan *et al.,* 1965, 1969a, b). *Pasteurella pneumotropica* is generally accepted as a causal organism of murine pneumonia and this was found in the lungs of sick mice. The other recurring condition was diarrhoea affecting young litters. Faecal specimens taken revealed the presence of *Proteus* species in up to 12% of animals. It must be remembered that the diarrhoea may have been viral in origin but no tests were undertaken to determine whether viruses were present.

The constant testing of both healthy and sick mice proved very useful in establishing the microbiological status of the colony: when this information became available, mice could be culled in a rational way so that only healthy stock was used in providing the nucleus of mothers whose litters were to be transferred to the barrier unit by hysterectomy.

The data obtained from the examination of sentinel mice provided interesting information on the transmission of microorganisms and also the movement of microorganisms within a holding room. Sentinel mice were placed so that one box of mice was at the air inlet end of the room and another level with the air outlet. It was soon observed that the respiratory tract of mice close to the air inlet was colonized by a smaller

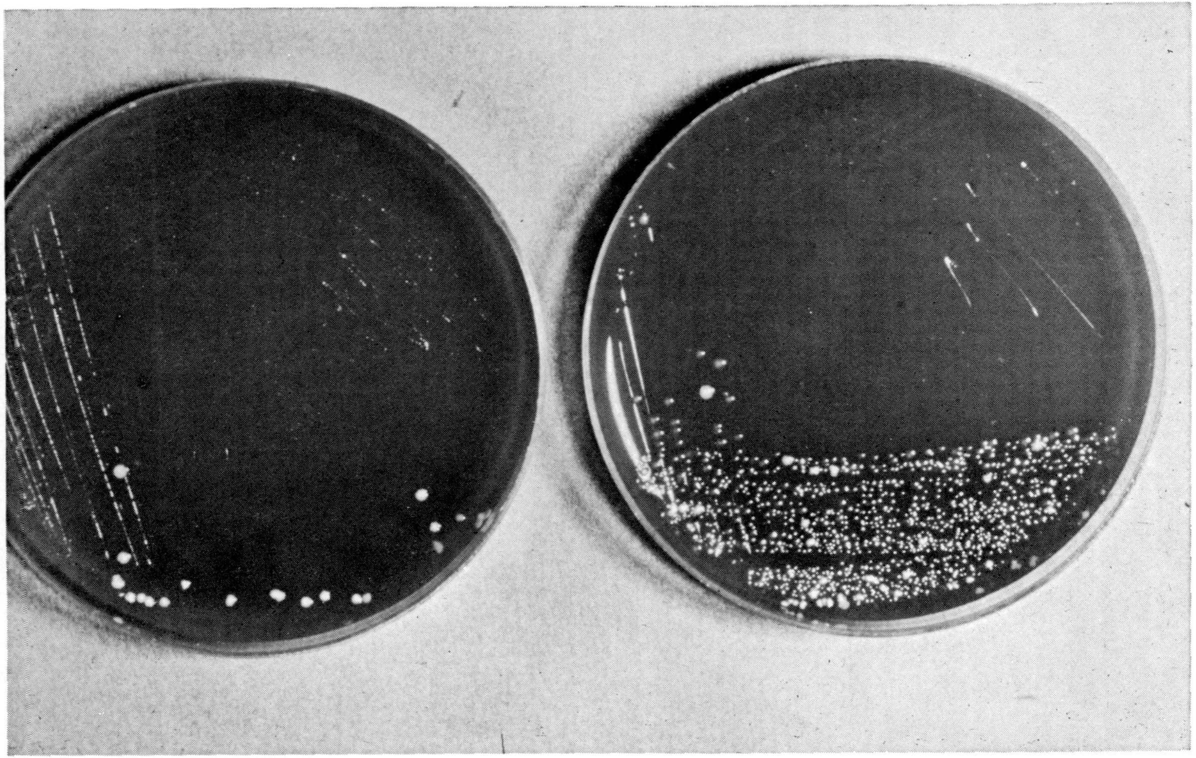

Fig. 9. Blood agar plates from throat swabs of sentinel mice. Left-hand plate taken from a mouse at the air inlet end of room showing less bacterial growth than the right-hand plate taken from the throat of a mouse by the air extract.

number of organisms than those at the other end of the room (Fig. 9). Also antibody levels to Sendai virus were significantly lower in mice at the clean end of the room. In addition to demonstrating the degree of infection within a room, these mice confirmed that those mice on the upper floor of the Animal House were colonized by less species of organisms than those on the lower floor.

It can be seen from Table 21 that the throats of mice in rooms located on the lower floor (2Y039-043, Level 2) were colonized by four or more species of organism, whilst those on the upper floor (3Y033-037, Level 3) were only colonized by two species of organism, *Pasteurella pneumotropica* and *Streptococcus* species. These results may be a purely random occurrence but they are more likely related to the breeding source and the type of experiments in progress on level 3 compared with the rooms on level 2. Only mice of barrier unit origin or category **** (Laboratory Animals Centre (LAC) accreditation scheme) were housed on level 3 and they were used for breeding and immunological experiments carried out without depletion of the host's defence mechanisms. In contrast, the mice on level 2 were supplied from sources outside the United Kingdom as well as commercial breeders in this country whose animals were of a lower category than **** in the LAC scheme. In addition to the poorer quality of animal on this floor they were used in experiments where modification of the mouse immune responses, for example by splenectomy, was frequently carried out. Undoubtedly, the impaired resistance to infection of many mice housed on level 2 combined with the fact that these mice were held in rooms stocked to a high density (3000 or more mice) accounted for their relatively poorer health. Similarly, *Mycoplasma* species and the ectoparasite, *Myobia musculi,* were only detected in mice from level 2.

Several interesting observations were obtained from the screening of sentinel animals. The transmission of *Mycoplasma* species from conventional mice to sentinels of barrier unit origin was found to take at least 3 weeks. Likewise, *Proteus* and *Klebsiella* species were first isolated after 4 weeks and the nematode *Syphacia obvelata* after 6 weeks. The mode of transmission of these organisms was probably the transference of faecal pellets which may occur when technicians' fingers become soiled whilst cleaning out the mice and this is a route of transmission that is generally disregarded. Contact between infected mice may also spread infection. The transmission of organisms by infected faeces was demonstrated by Sebesteny (1974) who showed the transference of intestinal flagellates between mice and rats by contact with soiled faeces.

Every batch of sentinel mice was tested for evidence of infection with Sendai virus but only a limited amount of testing was carried out for evidence of infection by Reo III, mouse hepatitis virus and Polyoma. All rooms were infected with Sendai virus although mice near the air inlet gave a lower titre on testing. No work was performed to study the rate of infection but it was found that the antibody titre rose over a 3 month period and then remained constant at $\frac{1}{256}$. Tyrell and Coid (1970) described a high antibody titre in rats 8 days after experimental infection and Tennant *et al.* (1966) reported 100% infection in mice accompanied by high antibody titres 25 days after exposure to Sendai virus. In view of their findings and the high titres obtained in conventional mice at this Centre, it would appear that a process of constant infection occurred.

Other workers have studied the mechanism of Sendai virus infection. Peace and Soave (1971) showed transmission of Sendai virus between conventional mice and mice of germ free origin, within 6 weeks of their being held together in a room. van der Veen *et al.* (1974) demonstrated transmission but they were unable to isolate the virus from nasal secretions. Their results suggested that once infected, a mouse was likely to resist further challenge, but an acutely infected mouse could transmit virus in aerosol form. At this Centre new mice enter each room weekly and therefore it would appear that these mice become infected and then are themselves responsible for infecting the next batch of mice. It would appear that within a conventional colony, Sendai virus is likely to be endemic; Poiley (1970) showed that only one colony out of six examined, was free from Sendai virus infection during the period "fourth quarter of 1967 to the second quarter of 1969". The only practicable system of control is to breed mice and conduct experiments behind efficient barriers but this severely limits access of research workers to their animals.

The other viruses, Reo III and mouse hepatitis virus, were not found in any batches of sentinel mice examined and it was therefore concluded that the Animal House was free from infection with these viruses. Polyoma virus was only found in one room (Table 22). There are conflicting opinions in the literature as to the prevalence of this virus. Parker *et al.* (1965) stated that Polyoma was commonly found in laboratory mice, whereas Poiley (1970) found no evidence of Polyoma infection in six centres tested. The source of the infection in the one room was not ascertained. Mice had entered the room after issue from the barrier unit, which was known to be free from infection, and also from the USA and Europe. It appeared therefore that the infection originated from one or both of the two latter sources.

Finally, the examination of sentinel mice from the infected suite revealed some interesting results when compared with the other areas. The rate of isolation of *Streptococcus* species was comparable with other areas but the rate of isolation of *Pasteurella pneumotropica* was significantly lower. By experiment (see Chapter 6) it was shown that mouse throats were quickly colonized by *Streptococcus* species when mice from the barrier unit were placed in conventional rooms, whereas colonization by *Pasteurella pneumotropica* occurred slowly. It was therefore presumed that animals issued from the barrier unit were colonized by *Streptococcus* species whilst held in the Animal House for some hours before being placed in the infected suite. Once inside the suite, the system of barriers used to contain infectious organisms prevented the entry of *Pasteurella pneumotropica* and hence the mice were not colonized by this organism. Sentinel mice placed in the room within the suite where work was in progress in isolators with Polyoma virus, *Mycoplasma pulmonis* and *Pasteurella pneumotropica* did not show infection with any of these organisms indicating that the isolator filters were efficient.

It was noticed that the numbers of organisms isolated from mouse throat samples was reduced following routine repainting of each conventional holding room but rose to original values 2 months after stock was returned to rooms. Furthermore, the number of species of bacteria recovered from each room has fallen as more homebred animals have been issued to them from the barrier unit.

Mice examined at the request of research workers were either ill, or alternatively, healthy but providing unexpected results in experiments. Whenever possible, the research worker was consulted to provide the background on the type of experiment in progress so that suitable and relevant tests could be carried out on the animal.

When the Animal House was first opened many research workers' mice were infested with ectoparasites. The advancing alopecia, sores and scabs seen on these mice resulted in many requests for laboratory help. Approximately 25% of mice examined on behalf of research workers were infested. Bacteriological culture of swabs taken from sores usually resulted in the growth of *Staphylococcus aureus* together with commensal enteric organisms. Ectoparasite infestation has been a problem encountered by research workers at this Centre (see Chapter 7).

Other conditions were encountered as isolated outbreaks or individual cases. On several occasions, mice were found to be suffering from eye infections. In these cases, the animals presented with increased lachrymal secretion, and *Pasteurella pneumotropica* was subsequently isolated from swabs taken from the affected eyes (Needham and Cooper, 1975). In one isolated incident, mice were examined in which the only clinical finding was a tail lesion resembling "ring tail" in rats (Fig. 10). 17 mice were affected and from 12 of these *Staphylococcus aureus* could be cultured

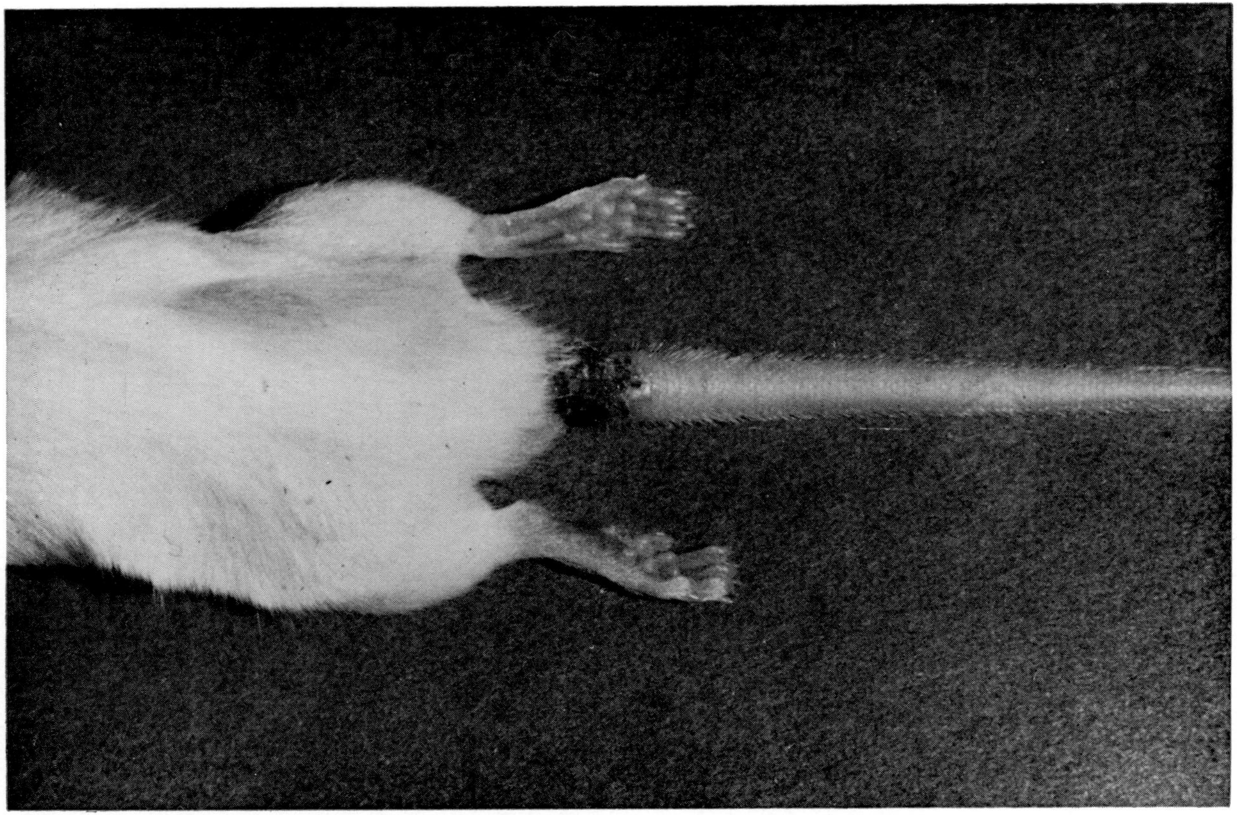

Fig. 10. Ringtail affecting a mouse.

from the lesion. Whilst no definite diagnosis could be made the cases occurred in one room in which it was known that the relative humidity had dropped suddenly from 60% to 40%. Such changes in humidity are known to predispose "ring tail" in rats. Mice were occasionally presented with clinical symptoms of respiratory illness; *Pasteurella pneumotropica* was often isolated from the lungs of these mice together with *Mycoplasma* species and the serum usually yielded a high titre against Sendai virus. It was felt likely that the combination of all three agents rather than one specific agent was responsible for the illness.

Mice examined in an attempt to explain unexpected experimental results often yielded inconclusive results. Some workers reported that abnormal immunoglobulin levels were being obtained from control animals, and when mice were examined they were found to have a severe ectoparasite burden which may have been responsible. On two occasions, separated by 12 months, a worker reported a failure to culture mouse macrophages *in vitro*, but extensive testing of his donor mice failed to reveal any good reason for this. However, on the second occasion the worker himself found that a change in the batch of serum used in the culture medium resulted in a perfect macrophage culture. In a further case, unexpected deaths during an experiment were traced to the original inoculum which was contaminated with bacteria.

In retrospect, feed back of information from scientists using the animals has proved the least valuable in establishing the health status of the colony. Perhaps this is not surprising in view of their tendency to blame the animals as soon as experiments fail, and the very complex interaction between their experimental protocol and the immunological status of the animal.

Conversely, animals examined on arrival at this Centre from commercial suppliers did provide some valuable data. As it was necessary to purchase animals, it was essential that an examination should be carried out as soon as possible after delivery. Table 24 shows the results obtained and it will be seen that 30% of throats and 5% of lungs were colonized by *Proteus* species. This was an isolation rate higher than any recorded in other groups of mice. This was surprising considering that the majority of mice purchased were category **** (LAC accreditation scheme). The significance of this finding was not determined. Flynn *et al.* (1956) isolated *Proteus mirabilis* from mice throats from 9 out of 11 suppliers, although the significance was not discussed. Other workers have reported work with *Proteus* species including the isolation of *Proteus mirabilis* from the organs of clinically sick mice (Jones *et al.*, 1972), and Miles (1951) reported varying pathological states when mice were infected with different strains of *Proteus vulgaris*. It was assumed that the presence of this organism in throats was probably due to the ingestion of faeces. Most suppliers did not include food whilst animals were in transit, so mice remained in transport boxes for up to 24 h in which time it is likely that faeces were ingested. A further unexpected isolate from category **** mice was *Pasteurella pneumotropica* as the presence of this organism is only acceptable in the lower grade category *** mice (LAC accreditation scheme). This was felt to be a significant isolate and one supplier was contacted with these results. After an initial reluctance to accept the microbiological findings it was discovered that animals of all categories were carried in one van. The transport boxes used did not incorporate any filters and hence in the relatively low air volume inside the van, susceptible animals were probably exposed to infection by aerosol inhalation. In fact, when the same supplier sent three batches of mice in filtered boxes *Pasteurella pneumotropica* was not isolated. The presence of *Mycoplasma* species in mice from one source, ectoparasites from another and large numbers of *Syphacia obvelata* in mice from a third supplier precluded further purchases from those sources.

The screening of suppliers may be compared with that carried out by the Laboratory Animals Centre. The Clinical Research Centre has the advantage of being able to screen a few suppliers several times a year and the supplier does not know that the animals are being examined. The LAC however screens many centres and can only sample each source twice a year when the supplier is asked to send six animals to the LAC.

The failure to isolate organisms from the disinfectant footpads in the infected suite was expected because of the well-known bacteriocidal action of chloros. Further, all staff entering the suite wore clean plastic overshoes so that possible contamination of these pads by large numbers of organisms on footwear was eliminated. It was felt that the direct sampling of the disinfectant pads with a blood agar plate was a valid technique as any residual chloros on the plate soon evaporated in the incubator.

It had been assumed that the detergent used in the cage wash ("Stretonite", Brentchem Ltd, London) together with the steaming process at the end of the wash would be sufficient to thoroughly clean the boxes. However, the preliminary experiment showed this to be a false assumption. There are many possible reasons for this failure and further experiments are planned to investigate these fully, but it is of value to discuss some of the main points. First, the detergent used is stated to be a sanitizing detergent. Investigations showed that the quantity of detergent used each day was not accurately measured into the tank at the start of the cleaning cycle. Furthermore, as water was lost, the level was automatically topped up so that the detergent was diluted, possibly to an ineffective level. Secondly, the temperature variation was seen to correlate with the number of organisms recovered. When the tanks remained at a low temperature a greater number of organisms were isolated. Thirdly, it was noticed that with the large number of boxes washed each day (1200 approximately) boxes were pushed through the machine faster than the conveyor speed, in an effort to save time. This obviously meant that boxes were not exposed to the detergent or the steam for the correct length of time. Also, again when time was short the boxes were not always thoroughly cleaned of bedding and faeces so that a large quantity of foreign material was introduced into the detergent tank.

The cage washing area presents an obvious weak link in preventing dissemination of pathogens and parasites within the Animal House. Ideally, all cages and rodent boxes should be thoroughly cleansed and sterilized.

6

Experimental Investigations in Conventionally Housed Mice

Introduction

Experiment 1: Colonization of Mouse Throats

The throat flora of sentinel mice was shown to be *Pasteurella pneumotropica*, and *Streptococcus* species (Table 21, Chapter 5). When sentinel mice were initially issued from the barrier unit, the throat flora consisted of only one organism, *Staphylococcus aureus*. However, when these mice were sampled after 1 month in conventional rooms, the staphylococcus was absent, apparently replaced by the other two organisms. It was decided to organize a short experiment to see at what time after issue the throat flora of the mice altered and which of the two organisms appeared first.

Experiment 2: Liver Infections in Apparently Healthy Mice

Male TO/Crc mice were used as sentinel mice at many sites within the Animal House. Boxes of these mice were sampled over a period of 6 months and subjected to the microbiological screen already described (Fig. 1).

Some mice which were apparently healthy and showed no clinical signs of disease, when submitted for *post mortem* examination presented abnormal livers. The appearance of these livers from time to time gave cause for concern due to the possibility of the presence of hepatic disease such as Tyzzer's disease or murine hepatitis. The livers were of normal consistency, but were various shades of brown and mottled in appearance (Plates 1 and 2). They were all subjected to pathological examination. Concurrently with the investigations, Hale and Hill (1973) published work showing that apparently normal livers of healthy mice yielded *Lactobacillus* species. It was known that *Lactobacillus acidophilus* and *lactis* were present in the intestines of mice in the barrier unit and in view of this, a study was initiated to examine livers of such mice. Parallel to this study, the programme of screening of sentinel mice from conventional rooms was continued and all abnormal livers were examined. A preliminary report of this work was published (Green *et al.*, 1975).

Experiment 3: Difference in Infection Rates Between Male and Female Mice

Experiments have been described to compare the methods used for the bacteriological sampling of rodent lungs. (See Chapter 3). During these experiments it was observed that female mice were not as easily infected as male mice.

Bouley *et al.* (1974) published results of their work showing that it was more difficult to infect female mice than male mice when using an aerosol of *Pasteurella multocida*. Due to the similarities of the route of infection and the organism it was decided to try and duplicate the work of Bouley *et al.* (1974).

It was hoped that by using mice issued from the barrier unit, the information gathered would provide additional data on the colonization of these mice by microorganisms.

Experiment 1: Colonization of Mouse Throats

Materials and Methods

Animals

The mice used were male TO/Crc strain, 4 weeks of age and issued direct from the barrier unit. Four were placed in a polypropylene box with wood chip bedding. Two boxes were placed in each conventional holding room already housing many mice, and were situated one at each end of the room.

Methods

Three rooms were studied, one with a small number (2000) of category **** mice (Townsend, 1969) (room 3Y037), another with a high stocking density (3000) of category **** mice, some on immunosuppression (room 2Y043) and a room (2Y040) with a high stocking density (3750) of experimental mice including a large number of imported mice.

Throat swabs were taken from live mice. The animal was gripped firmly at the back of the head and picked up so that the body hung downwards. In this position the mouth opened. The throat was swabbed with a nasopharyngeal swab (Calgiswab ref. 62-150-15 A. R. Horwell, Kilburn High Road, London), care being taken to avoid touching the tongue or teeth. The swab was rubbed on to a blood agar plate which was incubated aerobically at 37°C for 18 h. The organisms present were identified by standard procedures.

In the first experiment, specimens were first taken 24 h after issue and then every 48 h, whilst in the second experiment, throat swabs were obtained immediately on issue and then every 48 h.

Results

The first organism isolated was *Streptococcus* species. This was isolated within 24 h of the mice being placed in the conventional holding rooms and by 7 days all mice yielded *Streptococcus* species (Table 25). When issued from the barrier unit, *Staphylococcus aureus* was isolated from the throats but it was noticed that in the majority of mice this organism was replaced by *Streptococcus* species after 3 days. After 7 days, *Pasteurella pneumotropica* was isolated from a small percentage of mice. The actual figure varied and depended from which room the mice had been obtained. At 10 days, no mice in the lightly stocked room (3Y037) were colonized by *Pasteurella pneumotropica* and only 25% at 25 days. This contrasted with the other two rooms where in one (2Y043) 62% were colonized at 21 days but only 25% in the other (2Y040) (Tables 25 and 26). In the presence of *Pasteurella pneumotropica,* the number of colonies of *Streptococcus* species obtained from throat samples was reduced.

Table 25

Experiment 1: isolation of organisms from mice

Days after issue	Organism, number of isolates and room number								
	S. aureus			*Streptococcus* sp.			*P. pneumotropica*		
	3Y037	2Y040	2Y043	3Y037	2Y040	2Y043	3Y037	2Y040	2Y043
1	6/8	5/8	5/8	5/8	2/8	4/8	0/8	0/8	0/8
3	5/8	2/8	5/8	8/8	8/8	4/8	0/8	1/8	0/8
6	3/8	1/8	4/8	8/8	8/8	4/8	0/8	1/8	0/8
8	3/8	0/8	2/8	8/8	7/8	8/8	0/8	6/8	2/8
10	1/8	0/8	1/8	8/8	6/8	8/8	0/8	6/8	2/8
13	1/8	0/8	1/8	8/8	4/8	8/8	0/8	6/8	2/8
15	1/8	0/8	1/8	8/8	4/8	8/8	0/8	6/8	2/8
17	0/8	0/8	1/8	8/8	4/8	8/8	0/8	6/8	2/8
20	0/8	0/8	1/8	8/8	4/8	8/8	0/8	6/8	2/8
21	0/8	0/8	0/8	8/8	4/8	8/8	0/8	6/8	2/8

Table 26

Experiment 2: Isolation of organisms from mice

Days after issue	Organism, number of isolates and room number								
	S. aureus			*Streptococcus* sp.			*P. pneumotropica*		
	3Y037	2Y040	2Y043	3Y037	2Y040	2Y043	3Y037	2Y040	2Y043
0	7/8	8/8	8/8	0/8	0/8	0/8	0/8	0/8	0/8
2	1/8	3/8	4/8	8/8	7/8	6/8	0/8	0/8	0/8
4	0/8	1/8	0/8	8/8	7/8	8/8	0/8	0/8	0/8
7	0/8	1/8	0/8	8/8	7/8	8/8	0/8	0/8	0/8
9	0/8	0/8	0/8	8/8	8/8	8/8	0/8	2/8	1/8
11	0/8	0/8	0/8	8/8	8/8	8/8	0/8	3/8	1/8
14	0/8	0/8	0/8	8/8	8/8	8/8	0/8	4/8	1/8
16	0/8	0/8	0/8	8/8	8/8	8/8	0/8	4/8	1/8
18	0/8	0/8	0/8	8/8	8/8	8/8	0/8	4/8	1/8
21	0/8	0/8	0/8	8/8	8/8	8/8	1/8	4/8	1/8
23	0/8	0/8	0/8	8/8	8/8	8/8	1/8	4/8	1/8
25	0/8	0/8	0/8	8/8	8/8	8/8	2/8	4/8	2/8

Discussion

It was known that the throats of most mice in the barrier unit were colonized by *Staphylococcus aureus* but that this organism disappeared from throats of sentinel mice by the end of 1 month in a conventional room. The experiments performed showed that throats were differentially populated very rapidly after mice were introduced to a new environment.

Within 7 days of issue *Streptococcus* species could be isolated from all mice, and in some cases the new dominant inhabitant was established within 3 days. At this stage *Staphylococcus aureus* was still present but in very much reduced numbers. The *Staphylococcus aureus* was known to be of human origin and the rapid replacement of this organism by *Streptococcus* species suggested that the staphylococcus was unable to compete with a streptococcus of animal origin.

After 7 days the first isolates of *Pasteurella pneumotropica* appeared and the numbers of colonized mice gradually increased. It was found that over a long period of time (8 months) *Pasteurella pneumotropica* became the dominant organism replacing the *Streptococcus* species.

The speed with which this differential colonization occurs in mouse throats probably depends on several factors such as the stocking density of the room and the number of air changes per hour. As all the rooms used in the two experiments were force ventilated and the air changed 10–12 times each hour, it was assumed that the stocking density of each room was responsible for the different rate of colonization. Samples taken from mouse throats in the most densely stocked room (2Y040) revealed the presence of *Pasteurella pneumotropica* in approximately 50% of animals by day 10. In the other less densely stocked rooms only 25% of throats were colonized by day 20.

The knowledge gained by this experiment proved useful when allocating room space to research workers. On several occasions it was decided to place mice, to be used for immunological experiments or to act as donors of macrophages, in a room with only a small number of mice so that the animal's microbiological status did not substantially alter over a period of 1 month after issue from the barrier unit.

Experiment 2: Liver Infections in Apparently Healthy Mice

Materials and Methods

Animals

Two groups of mice from conventional rooms were examined. The first group was made up of 20 sentinel mice in which abnormal livers were observed at *post mortem* examination. The second contained 24 sentinel mice, obtained from six consecutive routine samples. A third group of mice was examined comprising 54 animals issued from the barrier maintained breeding unit.

Methods

Mice in the first group were subjected to the screening protocol already described (Fig. 1). When abnormal livers were observed (Plates 1 and 2), a lobe was cut and the freshly cut surface was rubbed on to two blood agar plates. One plate was incubated aerobically, the other anaerobically, both at 37°C for 18 h and a further 24 h if there was scanty or no growth. Organisms were then identified by standard methods. In addition, impression smears of the liver surface were made for staining by Gram's technique and Giemsa stain. A portion of the liver was obtained for histopathological examination and placed in 10% formal saline.

The mice comprising the other two groups were treated as described above, except that every liver was examined whether lesions were present or not.

Results

Lactobacillus species was identified as the organism present in some of the affected livers. It was isolated from eight mice issued from the barrier unit (Table 27(a), (b)) and 14 conventionally held mice yielded *Lactobacillus* species and five more yielded *Lactobacillus acidophilus* (Table 28(a), (b) and (c)).

Serological tests performed to test for the presence of mouse hepatitis virus indicated that all mice were free from infection (Tables 29(a), (b)).

The organism proved difficult to culture and grew on blood agar giving a colony of only 1 mm diameter. On several occasions the organism grew anaerobically but not aerobically. Normally the organisms

Table 27

(a) Experiment 2: barrier unit mice examined

Strain	Age and sex	Number examined	Liver		
			Gross appearance	Gram stain	Organism and number of isolates
TO/Crc	Adult M	15	Normal	—	2/15 *Lactobacillus* sp.
	10 week M	1	Brown mottled	—	No isolates
	8 week F	1	Brown mottled	—	*Lactobacillus* sp.
CBA/H-T6 Crc	3 week F	3	Normal	2/3 +ve rods	2/3 *L. acidophilus*
	3 week M	3	Normal	3/3 +ve rods	2/3 *L. acidophilus*
	Adult M	6	Normal	5/6 +ve rods	No isolates
	6 week M	6	1/6 Brown mottled	5/6 +ve rods	No isolates
	Adult F	1	Brown mottled	—	No isolates

(b) Experiment 2: barrier unit mice examined

BALB/cCrc	3 week M	3	Normal	3/3 +ve rods	No isolates
BALB/cCrc	3 week F	3	Normal	3/3 +ve rods	No isolates
BALB/cCrc	11 week M	3	Normal	2/3 +ve rods	1/3 *L. acidophilus*
BALB/cCrc	Adult F	3	Normal	1/3 +ve rods	No isolates
BALB/cCrc	Adult M	3	Normal	—	No isolates
BALB/cCrc	Adult F	3	Normal	1/3 +ve rods	No isolates

M, male; F, female; —, not examined.

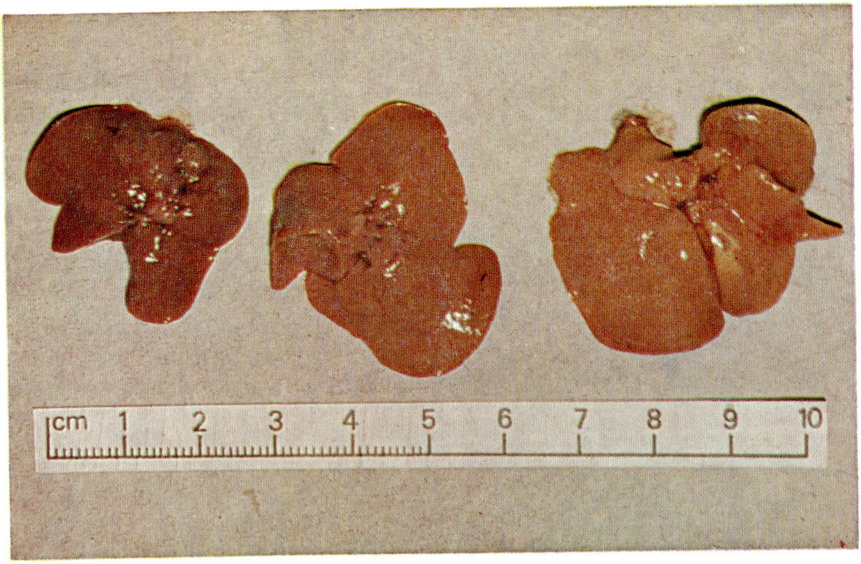

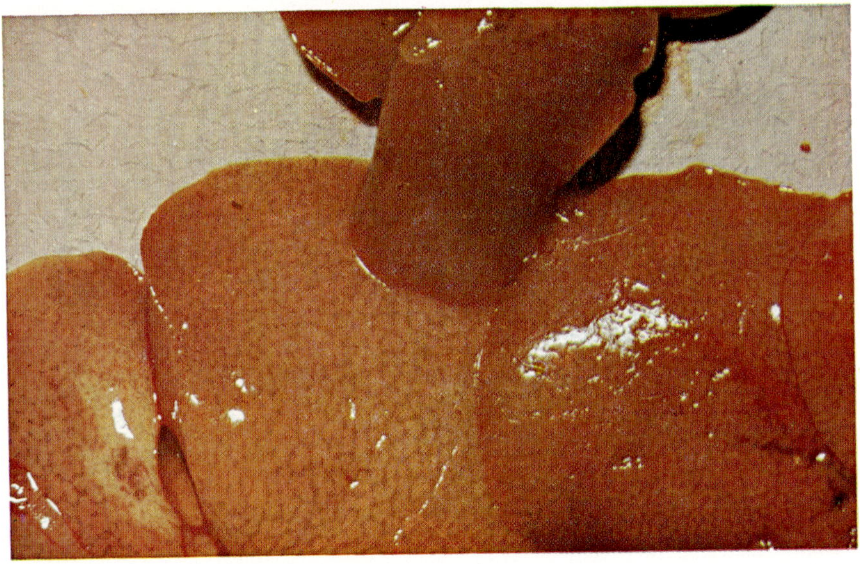

Plate 1. Mouse livers showing difference in size and degree of mottling. Left-hand liver from normal mouse, the other two showing an increase in size, pale colour and mottling.

Plate 2. Mouse livers showing mottling effect. Liver at top taken from normal mouse.

Table 28

(a) Experiment 2: mice examined after holding in conventional rooms

Strain	Age and sex	Number examined	Liver		
			Gross appearance	Gram stain	Organism and number of isolates
TO/Crc	8 months M	1	Brown mottled	—	No isolates
TO/Crc	12 weeks F	1	Brown mottled	—	*Lactobacillus* sp.
TO/Crc	9 weeks M	1	Brown mottled	—	*Lactobacillus* sp.
TO/Crc	14 weeks M	1	Brown mottled	—	Gram +ve rods
TO/Crc	18 weeks M	2	Brown mottled	—	2/2 *L. acidophilus*
TO/Crc	30 weeks M	1	Brown mottled	+ve rods	Gram +ve rods
TO/Crc	17 weeks M	1	Brown mottled	+ve rods	Gram +ve rods
TO/Crc	33 weeks M	1	Brown mottled	—	*Lactobacillus* sp.
TO/Crc	21 weeks M	1	Brown mottled	—	*Lactobacillus* sp.
TO/Crc	27 weeks M	1	Brown mottled	+ve rods	Gram +ve rods
TO/Crc	10 weeks F	1	Brown mottled	—	*Lactobacillus* sp.

M, male; F, female; —, not examined.

Table 28—*contd.*

(b) Experiment 2: mice examined after holding in conventional rooms

Strain	Age and sex	Number examined	Liver: Gross appearance	Liver: Gram stain	Liver: Organism and number of isolates
TO/Crc	21 weeks M	4	2/4 Brown mottled	—	1/4 *Lactobacillus* sp.
TO/Crc	21 weeks M	4	3/4 Brown mottled	—	3/4 *Lactobacillus* sp.
TO/Crc	9 weeks M	4	Normal	3/4 +ve rods	2/4 *Lactobacillus* sp.
TO/Crc	10 weeks M	4	Normal	2/4 +ve rods	No isolates
TO/Crc	11 weeks M	4	Normal	1/4 +ve rods	1/4 *L. acidophilus*
TO/Crc	24 weeks M	4	2/4 Brown mottled	2/4 +ve rods	2/4 *L. acidophilus*

(c) Experiment 2: mice examined after holding in conventional rooms

Strain	Age and sex	Number examined	Liver: Gross appearance	Liver: Gram stain	Liver: Organism and number of isolates
CD1	Adult F	1	Pale brown	—	Gram +ve rods
CD1	Adult M	1	Brown mottled	—	*Lactobacillus* sp.
CD1	Adult M	1	White lesions	—	*Lactobacillus* sp.
CD1	Adult F	1	White lesions	—	Gram +ve rods
AKR/Crc	Adult F	1	Brown mottled	+ve rods	Gram +ve rods
NZB/Crc	12 weeks F	1	Brown mottled	—	Gram +ve rods
NUDE	6 weeks M	1	Haemorrhagic	—	*Lactobacillus* sp.
CBA/CaCrc	4 weeks M	1	Brown mottled	—	*Klebsiella* sp.

M, male; F, female; —, not examined.

Table 29

(a) Experiment 2: antibody titre to mouse hepatitis virus in mice examined after holding in conventional rooms

Strain	Age and sex	Liver		Hepatitis titre
		Gross appearance	Organisms isolated	
TO/Crc	12 weeks F	Brown mottled	*Lactobacillus* sp.	1/10
TO/Crc	9 weeks M	Brown mottled	*Lactobacillus* sp.	1/5
TO/Crc	14 weeks M	Brown mottled	Gram +ve rods	1/20
TO/Crc	18 weeks M	Brown mottled	*L. acidophilus*	1/10
TO/Crc	30 weeks M	Brown mottled	Gram +ve rods	1/40
TO/Crc	17 weeks M	Brown mottled	Gram +ve rods	1/5
TO/Crc	21 weeks M	Brown mottled	*Lactobacillus* sp.	1/20
CD1	Adult F	White lesions	Gram +ve rods	1/5
CD1	Adult M	Brown mottled	*Lactobacillus* sp.	1/5
CD1	Adult M	White lesions	*Lactobacillus* sp.	1/5
NZB/Crc	12 weeks F	Brown mottled	Gram +ve rods	1/5

(b) Experiment 2: antibody titre to mouse hepatitis virus in mice issued from the barrier unit

TO/Crc	8 weeks F	Brown mottled	*Lactobacillus* sp.	1/5
CBA/H-T6Crc	Adult M	Normal	No isolates	1/5
BALB/cCrc	11 weeks M	Normal	*L. acidophilus*	1/5

M, male; F, female.

grew within 18 h, but in some instances further incubation was necessary to produce a sufficient number of colonies to allow identification to proceed. The organisms were identified according to Cowan and Steel (1966). In some cases it was not possible to identify the organisms and identification was limited to a Gram stain and morphological examination of the colony. These closely resembled the colonies identified as *Lactobacillus* species.

At no point in any of the three surveys were any organisms resembling those of Tyzzer's disease seen in smears and histological examination (Fig. 11) of all livers showed no gross pathological lesions although fatty degeneration was seen in a few cases.

Discussion

During the routine examination of sentinel mice, *Lactobacillus* species was isolated from livers that were brown and mottled in appearance. Samples taken from mice issued from the barrier unit also yielded this organism.

It is frequently assumed that abdominal organs of mice, including the liver, are sterile and the isolation of organisms from tissue is taken to indicate a disease process, although, in sheep and cattle, enteric organisms are regarded as saprophytes when isolated from livers. In view of the implications of the presence of this organism within mouse livers it was decided to investigate the condition. Also, it was debated whether the presence of this bacterial species may have predisposed either Tyzzer's disease or viral hepatitis.

Although Tyzzer published a report in 1917 of a condition found in the Japanese Waltzing Mouse, the causative organism still has to be grown on artificial media. For this reason diagnosis must rest on clinical and histological methods (Fig. 12). Diarrhoea is often associated with the disease and macroscopically there are opalescent pale grey nodules on the liver. A Gram stain should reveal clusters of thin long negative rods which may also be demonstrated by Giemsa stain. It was observed that none of the livers in this survey resembled the classical description but it was thought possible that the histopathological changes observed might be a precursor to classical Tyzzer's disease.

Impressions smears were made of the livers after removal from the animal for staining with Giemsa and Gram's technique. All livers in this study were fixed in formol saline, processed, and sections were stained with Gram's stain and haematoxylin and eosin. All smears and sections were carefully viewed but no Gram-negative rods were seen apart from

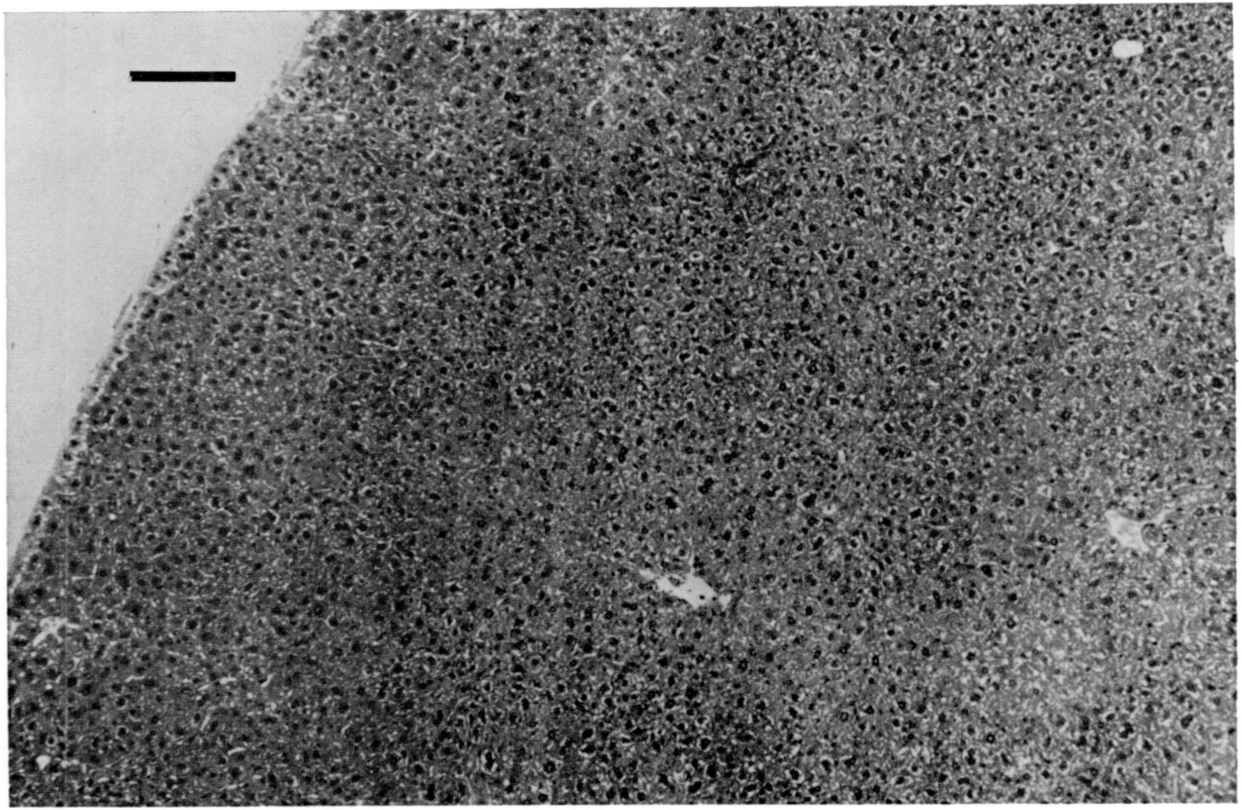

Fig. 11. Mouse liver taken from a severely mottled liver showing no pathological changes. Coles haematoxylin and eosin. Line represents 500 μm.

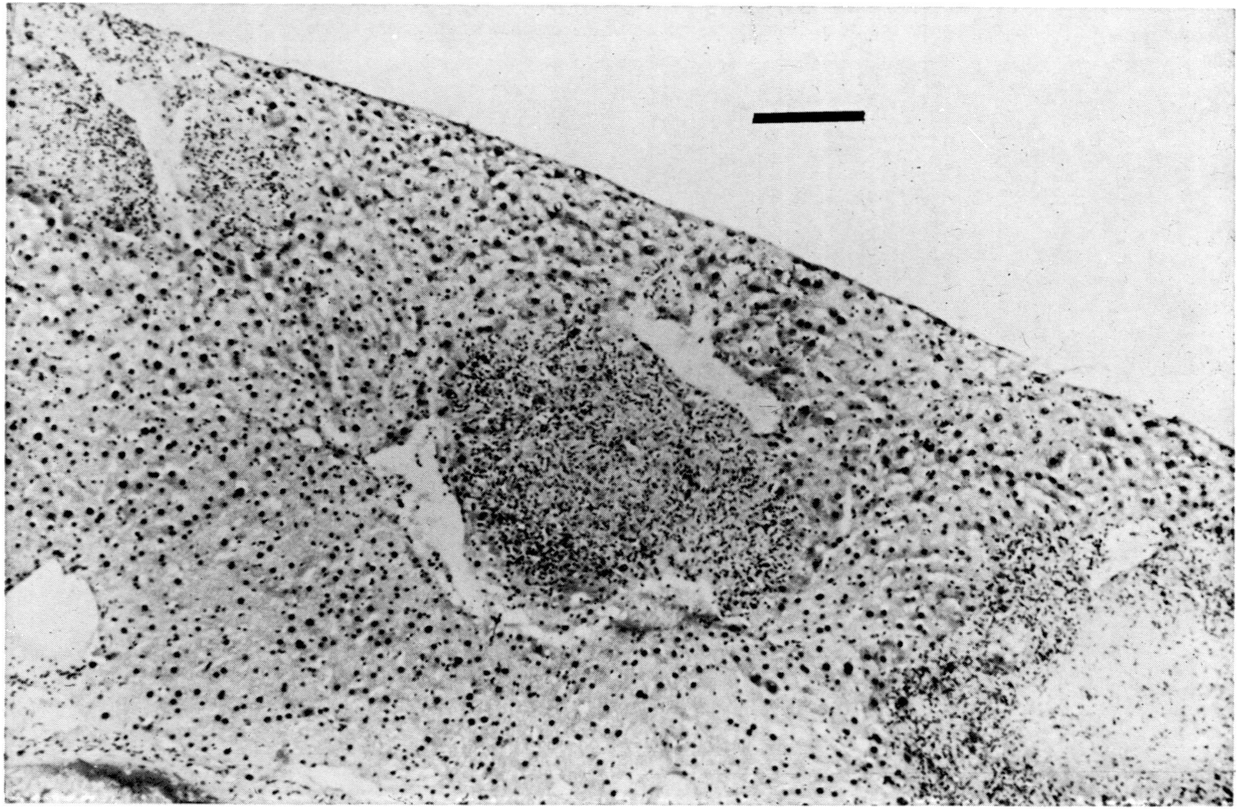

Fig. 12. Mouse liver from a case of Tyzzer's disease showing necrotic lesions. Coles haematoxylin and eosin. Line represents 500 μm.

one case which yielded *Klebsiella* species although thick Gram positive rods were observed in great number in many affected livers.

Murine hepatitis, which is present in many colonies as a latent viral infection, was considered as a possible cause of the liver abnormalities. However, the classical haemorrhagic lesions (Blackmore *et al.*, 1972b) (Fig. 13) were absent. It was decided that to exclude this disease, sera should be tested for antibodies. Arrangements were made with a commercial laboratory and 14 sera were examined, but these tests showed that none of the affected mice had antibodies to mouse hepatitis virus.

Lactobacillus was consistently isolated from the affected livers. This organism, although frequently isolated, was not necessarily associated with histological changes in the livers. Similarly, the appearance of Gram positive rods in Gram stained impression smears did not necessarily result in the isolation of *Lactobacillus* species on culture; perhaps this was because the organism proved very difficult to culture. In several cases small colonies were obtained which grew poorly in biochemical test sets so that identification could not proceed beyond colonial morphology and Gram stain result. However, morphologically these colonies resembled *Lactobacillus*. The failure to successfully culture greater numbers of these organisms may have been due to the medium used (blood agar)—and it is possible that the results would have improved if tomato juice agar had been used. Anaerobic culture was attempted in contrast to Hale and Hill (1973) and did result in the isolation of *Lactobacillus* species.

The role of *Lactobacillus* species in the liver perenchyma must remain speculative. It was thought likely that the organism reached the liver via the bile duct as it was known that *Lactobacillus acidophilus* and *lactis* had been given to the breeding stock in the initial reassociation mixture. *Lactobacillus acidophilus* appeared to be more hepatotrophic than *lactis*.

Experiment 3: Difference in Infection Rates Between Male and Female Mice

Materials and Methods

Animals

The mice used were all issued from the barrier maintained breeding unit and were placed in an isolator for the duration of each experiment. They were issued in four groups, (1) 36 male and 36 female TO/Crc mice at 8 weeks of age, (2) 36 male 5-week-old and 36 female 7-week-old TO/Crc

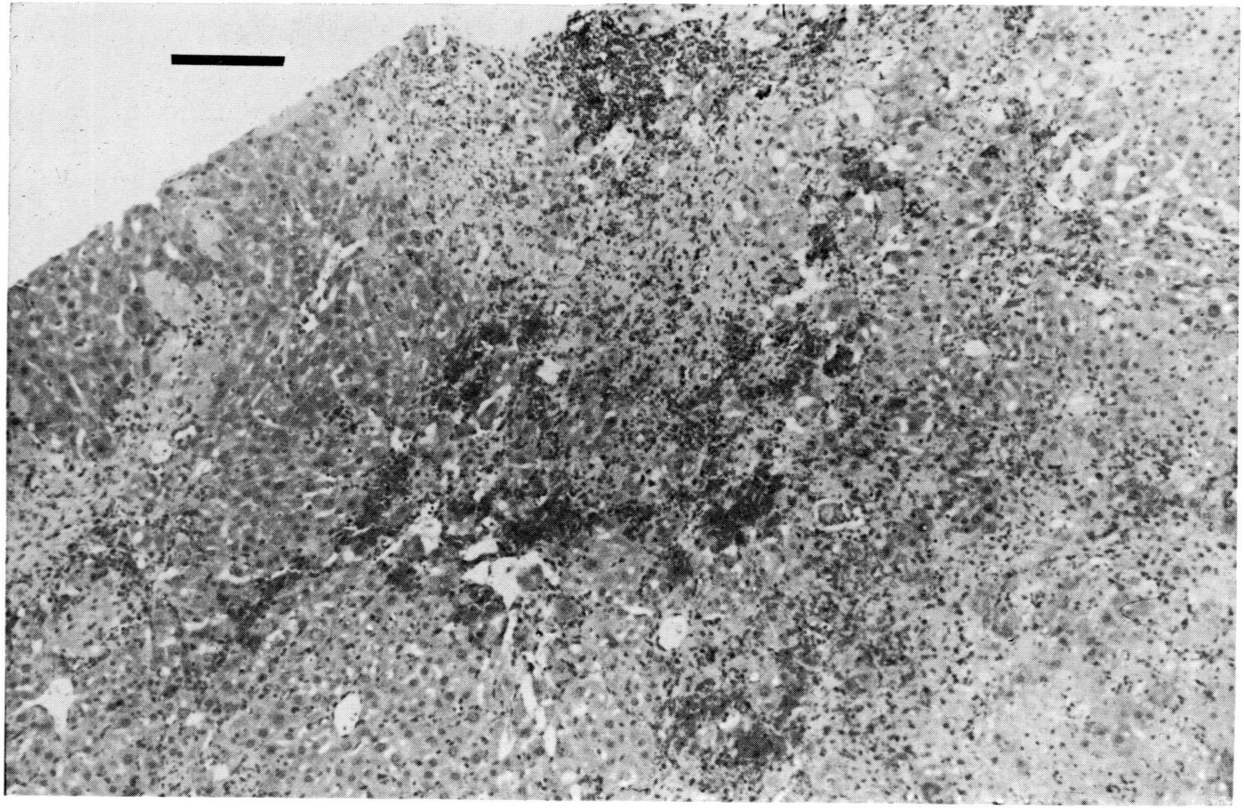

Fig. 13. Mouse liver from a case of murine hepatitis showing a lesion and areas of haemorrhage. Coles haematoxylin and eosin. Line represents 500 μm.

mice, (3) 36 male and 36 female BALB/c Crc mice at 8 weeks of age and (4) 36 male 5-week-old and 36 female 6-week-old BALB/c Crc mice. Groups (2) and (4) were issued with the weights of each sex approximately equal.

Organism

The organism used was *Pasteurella pneumotropica* isolated from a mouse throat and for use was cultured on blood agar for 18 h before being suspended in phosphate buffered saline.

Methods

In group 1, 36 male and 36 female 8-week-old TO/Crc mice were lightly anaesthetized under ether and were inoculated intranasally by placing drops of the organism suspension on the external nares. Each mouse received approximately 1×10^3 organisms in 0·1 ml of suspension. After 3 days, 12 mice of each sex were killed with an overdose of sodium pentobarbitone. Each animal was secured in dorsal recumbency and the thorax opened with aseptic precautions. The diaphragmatic lobe was cut and the cut surface was rubbed on to a blood agar plate which was incubated at 37°C for 18 h aerobically. The plates were read qualitatively for the presence of *Pasteurella pneumotropica*. This technique was repeated on days 4 and 7 post inoculation. In addition six control mice were intranasally inoculated with saline solution and examined on day 4.

The experiment was repeated three times, on groups 2, 3 and 4.

Results

The culture of lungs showed that more male mice yielded isolates than female mice, in an approximate ratio of 2:1 in the case of inbred BALB/c Crc mice and 3:1 in outbred TO/Crc mice (Table 30). A small histological survey of 12 control animals and 20 experimental animals revealed only five definite cases of pneumonic change. These could not be related to the sex, the weight, or the strain of mouse. No pneumonic changes were seen in any of the control mouse lungs examined.

Table 30

Experiment 3: number of isolates of *Pasteurella pneumotropica* obtained from mice lungs following intranasal inoculation

Mouse strain	Sex	Age	Number of isolates
TO/Crc	M	8 weeks	25/36
TO/Crc	F	8 weeks	8/36
TO/Crc	M	5 weeks	16/36
TO/Crc	F	7 weeks	5/36
BALB/c Crc	M	8 weeks	15/36
BALB/c Crc	F	8 weeks	6/36
BALB/c Crc	M	5 weeks	14/36
BALB/c Crc	F	6 weeks	7/36

No isolates were obtained from any of the eight control groups of mice.
M, male mice; F, female mice.

Discussion

The experiments showed that male mice are more easily infected by intranasal inoculation than female mice. This finding confirmed the work of Bouley *et al.* (1974). Bouley and Stupfel (1970) published a review paper and listed possible reasons for this difference in infection rates. Three main reasons were suggested, one being the influence of specific sex hormones, another the difference between male and female respiratory rates and minute volumes, and lastly the effects of holding mice in different environments, for example at different stocking densities.

The difference in respiratory function and the hormonal differences are the factors to be considered when interpreting the experimental results here presented, as environmental factors were carefully standardized. Mice of different sexes but of the same age will have a wide range of weights, with in general the male mice being heavier (Table 31). Guyton (1947) published results of a study measuring respiratory volumes of laboratory animals. He claimed that mice of a bodyweight approximately 20 g, have respiratory minute volumes ranging from 11·1 to 35·8 cm^3 min^{-1}. He calculated from his experimental data that the respiratory volume can be determined from a formula 2·10 × (bodyweight in grammes)$^{\frac{3}{4}}$. It is obvious therefore that with a wide weight range within a single group of mice, respiratory volumes must vary greatly.

Table 31

Experiment 3: weights of mice used

Mouse strain	Sex	Age	Bodyweight (g) ± standard deviation
TO/Crc	M	8 weeks	31·3 ± 5·8
TO/Crc	F	8 weeks	21·9 ± 6·3
TO/Crc	M	5 weeks	25·0 ± 2·3
TO/Crc	F	7 weeks	23·2 ± 1·5
BALB/c Crc	M	8 weeks	25·6 ± 1·6
BALB/c Crc	F	8 weeks	20·5 ± 1·1
BALB/c Crc	M	5 weeks	20·5 ± 3·9
BALB/c Crc	F	6 weeks	17·9 ± 1·2

M, male mice; F, female mice.

In order to see whether the respiratory minute volume was responsible for the difference in infection rates, male and female mice were used of approximately the same weights, in an effort to standardize lung size within narrow limits. However, it was found that the results obtained indicated that twice as many male mice were infected in contrast with the findings of Bouley *et al.* (1974).

Bouley *et al.* (1974) used an aerosol method of inoculation in his experiments which, from the work of Guyton (1947) would be subject to a large factor of error due to the different respiratory volumes. In the experiments recorded here, direct inoculation was carried out by placing drops of culture on the external nares. As respiratory volume was not a variant, this showed that any difference in infection rates between male and female mice was probably due to the sex hormones.

7

Ectoparasites of Mice: Mange Mites and their Control

Introduction

The most serious and far reaching health problem involving conventionally housed experimental mice during the first 7 years after the Animal House opened, was severe acariasis which proved difficult to control. Many of the mice concerned have undergone procedures that moderate the host's defence mechanisms and it is worth recording that mites were first positively identified on mice that had undergone splenectomy. This together with some initial environmental problems when the Animal House was first commissioned encouraged the increase in mite infestation, which in turn seriously interfered with the experiments being undertaken.

Many centres keeping mice in large numbers appear to be subject to infestation with mites and lice which cause mange and debilitation. One survey reported the identification of five species of mites and one species of louse from mice at various centres in the USA (Flynn, 1955). The most commonly found mites are *Myobia musculi* and *Myocoptes musculinus* (Flynn, 1955; Gambles, 1952). The pathogenic significance of these mites is in doubt (Oldham, 1967; Owen, 1972), although there are reports (Heston and Deringer, 1948; Galton, 1963) of *Myobia musculi* causing chronic dermatitis which may have led to secondary amyloidosis with renal impairment. Constantine (1972) reported that, when housed in an infested colony, immunologically depleted mice showed a rapid increase in infestation to the detriment of experiments in progress. The literature agrees that there is a marked variation in strain sensitivity; that heavy infestations depress conception rates in breeding colonies and that the resulting chronic dermatitis with its associated alopecia (Fig. 14), irritation and ulcerating lesions, cause losses which interfere with long term studies.

The sites of infestation and pathogenesis observed in mice in the Clinical Research Centre Animal House were similar to those reported by Constantine (1972). Originally some groups of mice were infested with both species of mite but after an initial dipping programme only *Myobia musculi* was observed, with very heavy infestation occurring around the head (Figs 15 and 16) and neck. Unlike other workers (Gambles, 1952; Cook, 1953a) no clear sex susceptibility to either species of mite was seen. However, strain susceptibility was seen. With a large number of infested mice available, the opportunity was taken to study the rate of infestation and this work was completed before eradication procedures were instituted.

The interference with experimental work became so serious that some eradication measures had to be carried out as quickly as possible. The colony to be treated numbered approximately 22 500 mice including the conventional breeding unit with young mice and there was also a constantly changing population within every room. The agent or agents to be used had to be effective after only two treatments and be safe both for mice and personnel.

Various agents have been claimed to be effective for the control of mites. Cook (1953b) reported that *Myobia musculi* responded to dipping in a 1·4% aqueous solution of tetrathylthuiram monosulphide ("Tetmosol", Imperial Chemical Industries, Alderley Park, Macclesfield, SK10 4FT) whereas *Myocoptes musculinus* could be eliminated by dusting with benzene hexachloride, but this was ineffective against *Myobia*. "Aramite" (2-tert-butyl-phenoxyl isopropyl-2-chloro-ethyl sulphite) was said to clear mice of mites (Flynn, 1955); 2% Malathion (00-dimethyl dithiophosphate of diethyl mercaptosuccinate) used as a dip was recommended by Davis (1957) to eradicate *Myocoptes musculinus*: Madden *et al.* (1954) compared sulphur and "Lindane" (gamma benzene hexachloride) and concluded that effective control was achieved using sulphur alone. Unfortunately most of these measures were time consuming and unrealistic for a colony of the size to be treated.

As Tetmosol appeared to be the most effective acaricide, this was used to try and clear all the mice in the conventional colony with the exception of the breeding colony. The mice were dipped into a 2·5% solution, warmed to 37°C. This treatment rapidly cleared the colony of *Myocoptes musculinus* but only reduced the burden of *Myobia musculi*. This result differed from reports in the literature, and as it was necessary to

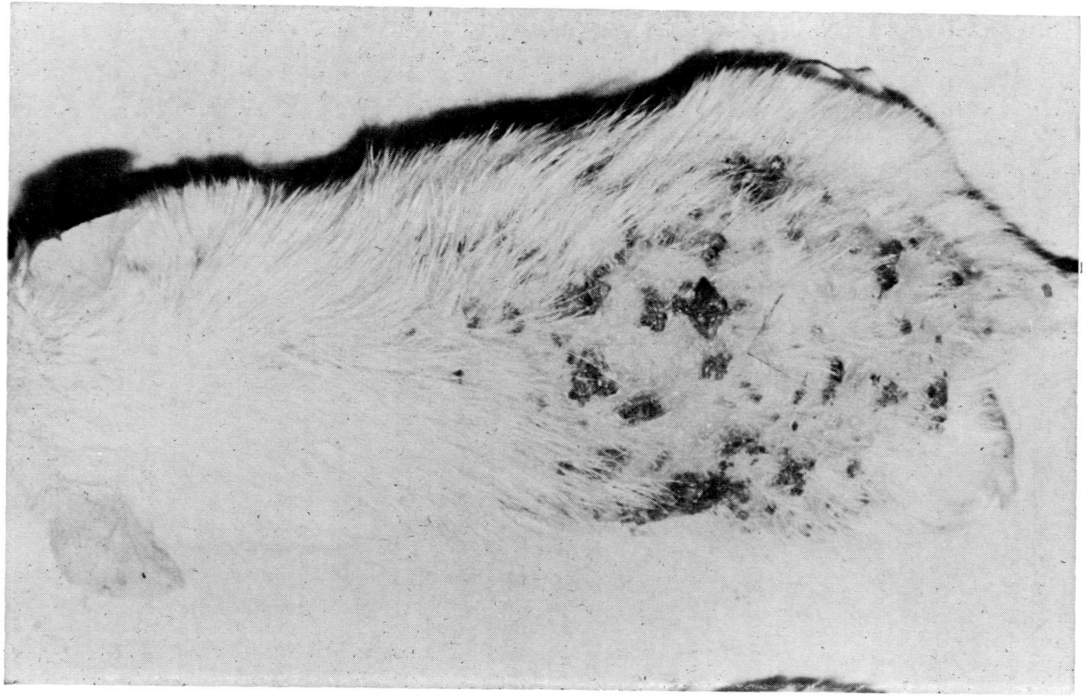

Fig. 14. Severely mite-infested mouse with alopecia and scabs.

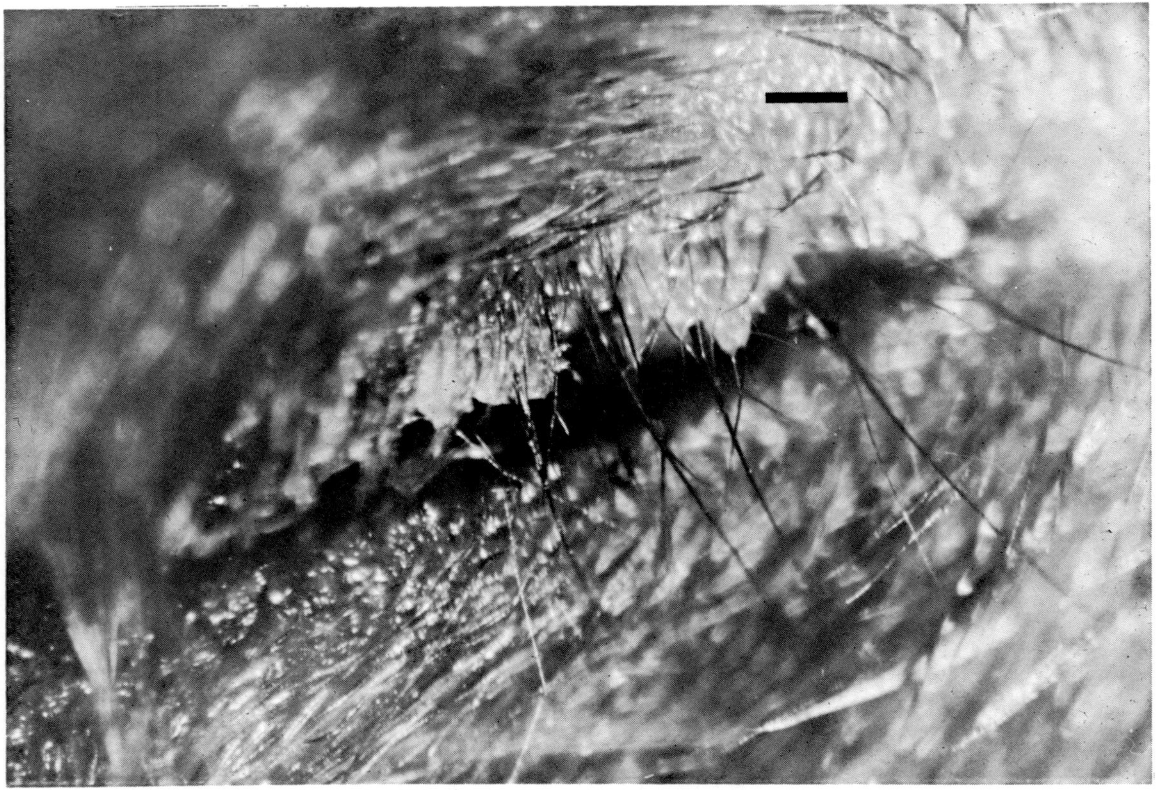

Fig. 15. *Myobia musculi* embedded on the eyelid of a mouse. Line represents 1 mm.

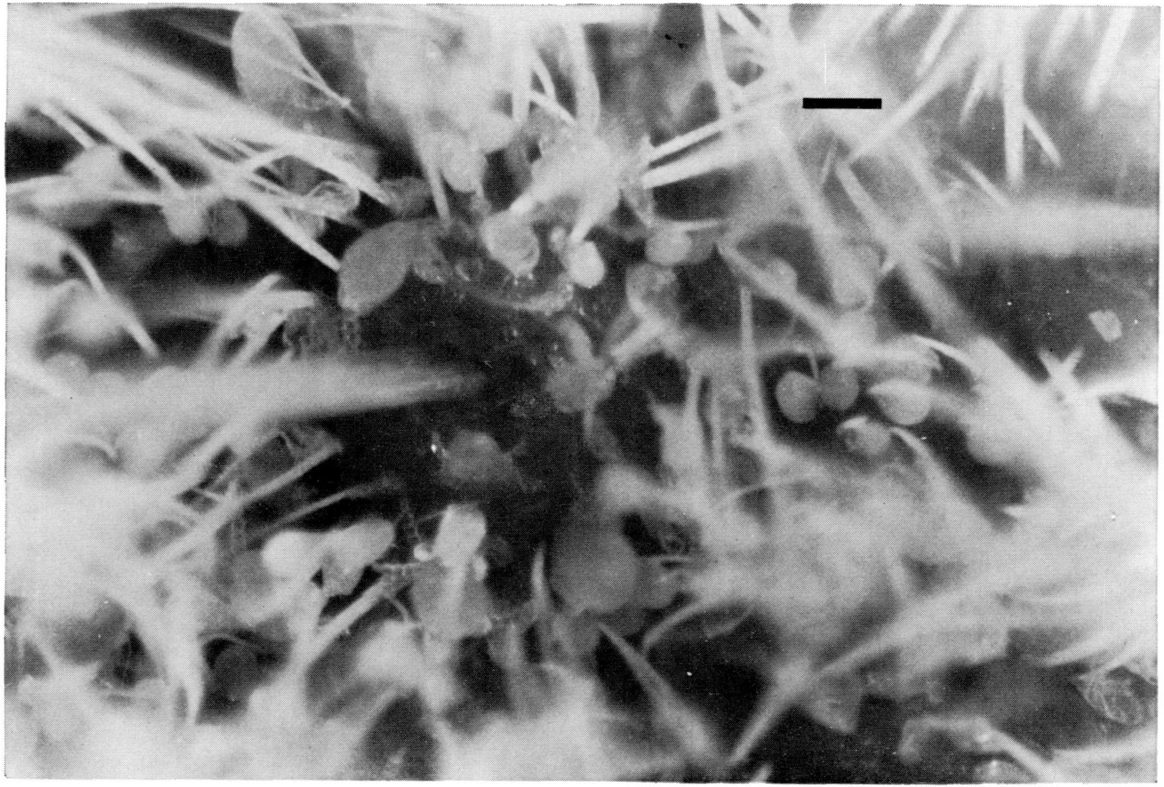

Fig. 16. *Myobia musculi* and ova on the muzzle of a badly infested mouse. Line represents 250 μm.

completely eradicate mites, it was decided to investigate several possible treatments in a systematic way.

A study was undertaken to compare Malathion, Tetmosol and benzene hexachloride (BHC). A further study was initiated using synergized pyrethrins (Green and Needham, 1974a) following a report (Constantine, 1972) detailing the successful treatment of acariacis with Pyractone (Bush Boake Allen Ltd, Blackhorse Lane, London, E17 5QP). However, the concentrations of the components of this product as recorded by Constantine, were unknown to the manufacturers and it was assumed that he was referring to Pyractone M429. It was decided to investigate the dose response of this product and also Pyractone M817 and hence arrive at a suitable dose. After the dose response experiments, work with Pyractone M817 was discontinued and it was considered worthwhile to see whether the components of Pyractone M429 acted as acaracides when used singly and also whether there was a toxic dose of the product. When these studies were completed the entire conventionally housed colony was treated with synergized pyrethrins (Super Decolourized Pyractone M429). However, mites reappeared after approximately 4 months and a third study was undertaken to test the effectiveness of flowers of sulphur (Green and Needham, 1974b).

The experiments which were carried out in order to deduce logical control measures are described in detail below.

Experiment 1: Rate of Infestation of Mice with *Myobiamusculi*

Materials and Methods

Animals

17 mite-free 1-year-old TO/Crc strain male and female mice were housed with two heavily mite infested mice on atapulgite clay bedding ("Sterolit", S. P. Usher Ltd, 46 Chandos Avenue, London) in a polypropylene box.

Methods

At the start of the experiment, the mice were examined under a × 20 viewing microscope whilst under light ether anaesthesia. The number of mites or ova present was noted and the mice were graded accordingly:

2 or less mites/ova per field, +
3–4 mites/ova per field, ++
5–6 mites/ova per field, +++
7 or more mites/ova per field, ++++.

The mice were viewed every 72 h for 9 weeks. They were cared for by conventional husbandry throughout the experiment.

Results

The mice were held for 9 weeks. After 4 weeks 25% had become infested. At 5 weeks 60% were infested and all were infested by 6 weeks (Table 32). The sudden rise in the degree of infestation coincided with the appearance of clinical cases of sinusitis.

Table 32
Experiment 1: rate of infestation of TO/Crc mice

Time in weeks	Number of mice with mites
1	3/17
2	3/17
3	3/17
4	4/17
5	10/17
6	17/17
7	17/17
8	17/17
9	17/17

Some female mice successfully raised litters during the experiment. It was observed that young mice did not become infested for 7 days following birth, but after this time infestation progressed steadily.

Experiment 2: Comparison of Tetmosol, Malathion and Benzene Hexachloride

Materials and Methods

Animals

6-month-old male or female TO/Crc strain were used and held in polypropylene boxes with atapulgite clay bedding. The animals were held under conventional conditions and allowed to breed and raise litters.

Agents

"Tetmosol" (tetraethylthiuram monosulphide) suspension as a 2·5% dip (Imperial Chemical Industries, Pharmaceuticals Division, Alderley Park, Macclesfield, SK10 4FT).

"Malathion" powder (00-dimethyl dithiophosphate of diethyl mercaptosuccinate) as a 2·5% dip (Cooper, McDougall and Robertson Ltd., Berkhamsted, Herts.).

Benzene hexachloride (BHC) suspension as a dip giving 0·625% active agent (Cooper, McDougall and Robertson Ltd).

Methods

The three agents were all used at the dosages suggested by previous workers, Malathion and Tetmosol each at 2·5% and benzene hexachloride at 0·625%. Groups of mice were dipped in the acaricide under test. Each solution was warmed to 37°C and held at this temperature; all mice were completely immersed, either by a single dip or by making them swim along a 1·2 m trough containing Tetmosol; whilst in the trough the animals were pushed under twice to ensure thorough wetting of the head. After treatment the mice were placed in clean boxes, with paper tissues to form a nest, and allowed to dry at room temperature (22°C). After 24 h clean wood chip bedding was added. 14 days after treatment, dipping was repeated. Once a week for 9 weeks after the initial treatment the mice were viewed and graded as already described. Any litters born after the first treatment were dipped with their parents when these were redipped.

Results

A strain difference in the degree of infestation was noted during this experiment. BALB/c Crc and AKR/Crc mice were always heavily infested, TO/Crc mice to a lesser degree, NZB/Crc and C57BL/10ScSnCrc only lightly infested and CBA/CaCrc and CBA/H-T6Crc rarely infested. No difference in the degree of infestation was found when male and female mice were compared.

When comparing known acaricides it was found that Malathion was totally ineffective (Table 33). Benzene hexachloride was found to be virtually ineffective with only one mouse successfully treated. Tetmosol at 2·5% proved relatively effective clearing all but two of the infested mice, although it made no difference whether the mice were dipped or forced to swim along a trough.

Approximately 10% of the mice died following treatment with these agents but mortalities were thought to be the result of fighting.

Experiment 3: Comparison of Synergized Pyrethrins

Materials and Methods

Animals

6-month-old male or female TO/Crc strain mice were used and held in polypropylene boxes with sterile wood chip bedding. The animals were held under conventional conditions and allowed to breed and raise litters.

Agents

"Super Decolourized Pyractone M429" (5% active pyrethrins synergized with 25% bucarpolate) (Bush Boake Allen Ltd, Blackhorse Lane, London E17 5QP).

Bucarpolate 25% emulsion (ester of piperonylic acid with the mono-u-butyl ether of diethylene glycol) (Bush Boake Allen Ltd).

"Pyractone M817" (8% active pyrethrins synergized with 64% piperonyl butoxide) (Bush Boake Allen Ltd).

Pyrethrins 25% emulsion (Bush Boake Allen Ltd).

Methods

The first investigations were set up to assess a dose response for Pyractone M429 and Pyractone M817. Pyractone M429 was diluted to give a solution of 0·25% active pyrethrins + 1·2% bucarpolate, which was double diluted to give a further three dilutions. Pyractone M817 was diluted to give an initial concentration of 0·25% pyrethrin + 2% piperonyl butoxide which was double diluted to give three further dilutions.

Table 33

Experiment 2: comparison of acaricides in mice

Acaricide	Mice starting trial	Mice with mites or eggs (days after first dip)								
		7	14[a]	21	28	35	42	49	56	63
Malathion 2·5%	20	20/20	20/20	20/20	20/20	20/20	20/20	20/20	20/20	20/20
Tetmosol 2·5% dip	20	18/20	12/18	2/16	2/16	2/16	2/16	2/16	2/16	2/16
Tetmosol 2·5% in trough	20	18/20	17/20	3/19	3/19	2/19	2/19	2/19	2/19	2/19
BHC 0·625%	10	4/10	4/10	3/9	6/9	7/9	7/9	8/9	8/9	8/9
Untreated control	20	20/20	19/20	19/20	19/20	19/20	19/20	19/20	19/20	19/20

[a] 2nd treatment; BHC, benzene hexachloride.

Groups of 10 mice were then dipped with a different dilution for each group and were afterwards placed in clean boxes with wood chip bedding. Dipping was repeated 14 days after the first treatment and the mice were then examined and the infestation graded over a 7 week period.

When the results of these investigations were known, it was decided to investigate the effect of pyrethrins and bucarpolate separately.

Pyrethrin was diluted to give concentrations of 0·125%, 0·06% and 0·03% and bucarpolate was diluted to give concentrations of 0·6%, 0·3% and 0·15%. Ten mice were used in each group, one group per dilution, each being dipped twice as before and then observed for 7 weeks.

The final investigation was a toxicity test using pyrethrin. Pyrethrin was double diluted from 0·5% to 0·03%. Ten mice were again used per dilution, the groups used for the two highest concentrations were dipped once only and the others were dipped twice at a 14-day interval.

At the end of each investigation the mice were killed and subjected to *post mortem* examination. The livers were removed for histological examination and particular attention paid to the degenerative changes.

Results

It was found that Pyractone M429 produced severe nervous signs at the highest dose used in the dose response investigation. Mice dipped in 0·25% active pyrethrins became hyperactive and nervous within 30 min of dipping and were killed. Those dipped in 0·125% pyrethrins showed a slight increase in activity but were normal within 24 h. The other groups did not show any signs of hyperactivity. Concentrations of 0·125% and 0·06% pyrethrin cleared the mice of mites (Table 34), but 0·03% pyrethrin did not.

Pyractone M817 was investigated in the same manner and at the same dilutions of active pyrethrins. In common with M429, nervous activity increased at the highest concentration and it was found that the fur of the mice could be easily pulled out. 0·125% pyrethrins cleared mice of mites but in contrast with M429, mice were not cleared by 0·06% (Table 35).

When the components of M429 were tested singly, pyrethrin, at a dilution likely to produce nervous side effects, did not clear mice of mites. Bucarpolate at the corresponding dilutions did not clear the animals of the ectoparasite (Table 36).

Due to the possibility of side effects with pyrethrins, pyrethrin was used in a toxicity test. Mice dipped in 0·5% and 0·25% developed

Table 34

Experiment 3: dose response to "Pyractone M429"

% pyrethrins + % bucarpolate	Mice starting trial	Mice with mites or eggs (days after first dip) 7	14[a]	21	28	35	42	49
0·25 + 1·2	10[b]	—	—	—	—	—	—	—
0·125 + 0·6	10	3/10	1/10	0/10	0/10	0/10	0/10	0/10
0·06 + 0·3	10	3/10	2/10	0/10	0/10	0/10	0/10	0/10
0·03 + 0·15	10	6/10	3/10	2/10	2/10	2/10	2/10	2/10

[a] 2nd treatment; [b] killed on day of treatment.

Table 35

Experiment 3: dose response to "Pyractone M817"

% pyrethrin + % piperonyl butoxide	Mice starting trial	Mice with mites or eggs (days after first dip) 7	14[a]	21	28	35	42	49
0·25 + 2·0	10[b]	—	—	—	—	—	—	—
0·125 + 1·0	10	5/10	2/10	0/10	0/10	0/10	0/10	0/10
0·06 + 0·5	10	4/10	4/10	1/10	2/10	2/10	2/10	4/10
0·03 + 0·25	10	6/10	5/10	3/10	3/10	3/10	3/10	4/10

[a] 2nd treatment; [b] killed on day of treatment.

Table 36

Experiment 3: effects of components of "Pyractone M429" used singly

Component %	Mice starting trial	Mice with mites or eggs (days after first dip) 7	14[a]	21	28	35	42	49
Pyrethrin								
0·125	10	2/10	2/10	2/10	2/10	2/10	2/10	2/10
0·06	10	6/10	6/10	6/10	8/10	8/10	8/10	8/10
0·03	10	8/10	8/10	8/10	8/10	8/10	8/10	8/10
Bucarpolate								
0·6	10	4/10	4/10	6/10	6/10	6/10	6/10	6/10
0·3	10	2/10	6/10	6/10	6/10	6/10	6/10	6/10
0·15	10	6/10	4/10	6/10	6/10	6/10	6/10	6/10

[a] 2nd treatment.

nervous signs within 10 min and were killed. Within 1 h, mice dipped in a dilution of 0·125% developed slight nervous signs which disappeared over 24 h. Dilutions of 0·06% and 0·03% did not produce any side effects.

Histological examination of livers from all treated mice revealed no abnormalities.

Experiment 4: Effectiveness of Sulphur Powder

Materials and Methods

Animals

The initial experiment was performed on 10 heavily infested 1-year-old AKR/Crc strain mice. The second experiment involved 32 adult NZB/Crc mice held one to a box with wood chip bedding.

Agent

Flowers of sulphur BP (Fison's Scientific Apparatus, Loughborough, Leicestershire).

Methods

Sulphur, as a powder, presented difficulties as to its mode of application. To overcome these difficulties, a perspex drum was designed (Green and Needham, 1974b) (Fig. 17).

The initial experiment involved 10 heavily infested 1-year-old AKR/Crc mice. They were treated in the drum in two batches of five. Sulphur powder was added taking care to break up any lumps. Each group was rotated in the drum for 15 revolutions changing the direction of rotation every three revolutions. This process was repeated after 14 days, each mouse being viewed as before over a period of 10 weeks.

The second experiment involved 32 adult NZB/Crc mice, one to a box. These mice were rolled one at a time, this being repeated on day 4, when a little sulphur was added to the wood chip bedding. On days 4 and 7 the mice were examined under a dissecting microscope.

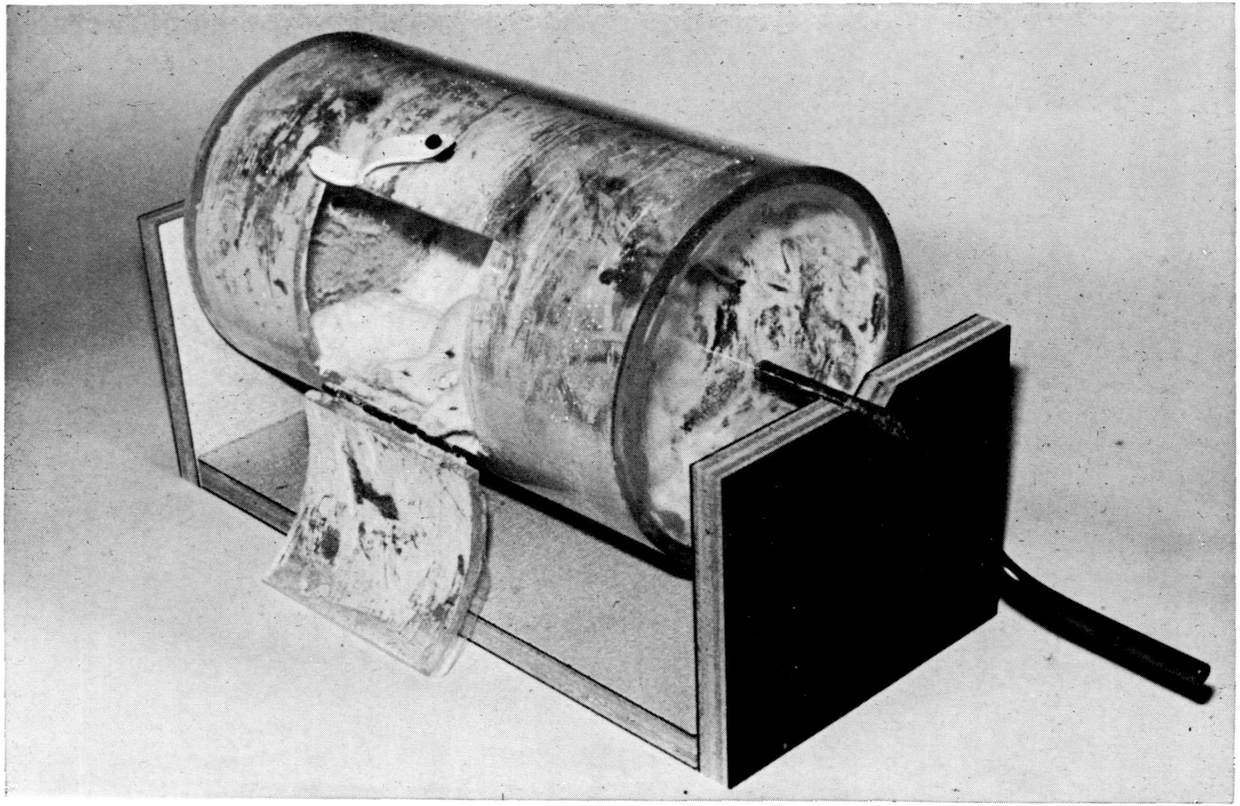

Fig. 17. Tumbler for sulphur treatment of mice.

Results

The mice treated with sulphur in the first experiment were cleared of mites 7 days after treatment. In the second investigation, only 60% of mice were cleared of mites 7 days after treatment, although it was observed that the alopecia was regressing.

Discussion

Throughout all the experiments, the infestation of each mouse was graded as already described. When selecting mice for use in an experiment, a count was performed of the number of mites present in each field under the microscope and only mice with more than 10 mites per field were used. During the course of experiments the particular agents in use were assessed by their ability to clear mice of mites and ova after two treatments.

The infestation rate experiment (experiment 1) showed that healthy mice can resist infestation for some time. When some mice developed sinusitis the rate of infestation increased dramatically. This clearly demonstrated the ability of the mite to rapidly multiply on debilitated mice and probably represents the mode of progressive build up in a mouse room. Within each room at this Centre there are between 3000 and 3500 mice at any one time. Many of these have depleted defence mechanisms and some are moved between boxes. Therefore infested mice may easily transmit mites to other mice within the room.

Young litters born to infested mice in this short experiment were observed and it was found that until the young were older than 7 days, no mites or ova were seen. This was almost certainly due to the lack of fur thus depriving mites of an attachment point. After 7 days the young were slowly infested, the degree of infestation increasing with the growth of fur. These observations led to the decision that a successful acaricide must be safe to use with mice as young as 7 days.

The comparison of acaricides (experiment 2) already in common use proved interesting in that the results obtained with Malathion and benzene hexachloride were very disappointing. Malathion was totally ineffective and benzene hexachloride was surprisingly ineffective at 0·625% considering its proven ability to treat acariacis in other species. Mice treated with benzene hexachloride that were apparently clear of mites 7 days after the second treatment became reinfested, finally resulting in a situation nearly as bad as before treatment was initiated. The two different methods of application of Tetmosol did not show any significant difference in effectiveness. As the dipping method was considerably easier to carry out, the other was discontinued. A 2·5% solution of Tetmosol was relatively effective, clearing all but two of the mice, and these retained a low grade *Myobia musculi* infestation of the eyelids (Fig. 16). The untreated controls remained heavily infested with advancing alopecia and sores.

It was decided after this experiment that Tetmosol was a suitable acaricide with which to start treatment of the infested rooms within the Animal House. The safety factor was good with no harmful effects seen on young mice. This dipping programme reduced the burden of *Myobia musculi* in all rooms treated and cleared the Animal House of *Myocoptes musculinus*.

Constantine (1972) reported very successful treatment with Pyractone and as mites still persisted in many rooms a series of investigations (experiment 3) were designed to find a suitable dose of Pyractone. Two Pyractone products were available and the results of the dose response of the mice to these has been recorded in Tables 34 and 35. A concentration of 0·06% active pyrethrin did not prove toxic, but only when synergized with bucarpolate in M429 was it an effective acaricide.

It was also observed that the properties of Pyractone M429 were more suitable for use as a dipping agent. M429 wetted a mouse more thoroughly than any of the previous acaricides studied, whereas Pyractone M817 was oily, did not wet the mice thoroughly and was difficult to suspend at the correct concentration in the dipping tank as it tended to form a layer on the surface of the water. This layer clung to the fur of mice as they were dipped. It was observed that when mice were killed because of toxic side effects, it was possible to pull the fur out easily only a few hours after treatment with M817, whereas with M429 the fur could not be removed and based on the experimental results it was concluded that work with M817 should be discontinued. However, the oily property of M817 has been found to make the product suitable for aerosol administration and Page (1974) reported the successful clearance of lice from guinea-pigs by this method. But, this mode of application was considered to be impractical in the holding rooms at this Centre.

The final investigations were a toxicity test and tests to see whether the components of M429 would act as an acaricide when used singly. The results of these tests have been recorded in Table 36. No toxicity with M429 was observed at the lowest dilution necessary to clear mites. The components of Pyractone M429 did not act as acaricides, demonstrating the synergistic nature of the two components.

At the conclusion of all the pilot trials it was decided that a large scale trial should be organized. A room with a large number of infested mice was selected and in the first trial half of the mice in the room were treated. The animals were dipped twice 14 days apart and they were viewed weekly for 7 weeks following the initial dip. The results are shown in Table 37, where it can be seen that mites were not eliminated. This was thought to be due to several possible factors; the most important was likely to be due to imperfect wetting. It was decided to dip the mice again, but to dip them in warm water to wet them, remove bedding and dust before dipping in the M429. This procedure was highly successful. Eight weeks after this third dip the entire colony within that room was dipped twice incorporating the same wetting procedure and the room was completely cleared of mites. There were no deaths amongst the 4500 mice.

Table 37

Grading of infestation of mice dipped in large scale trial with "Pyractone M429"

	Week after first dip							
Strain	0[a]	1	2	3	4	5	6	7
BALB/c Crc	++	+++	++	++	+	—	—	—
NZB/Crc	+	—	—	—	—	—	—	—
AKR/Crc	++++	+++	++	++	+	+	+	—
CBA/H-T6 Crc	—	—	—	—	—	—	—	—

[a] Day of first dip.
++++, 9 or more mites per field; +++, 6–8 mites per field; ++, 3–5 mites per field; +, 2 or less mites per field; —, no mites or eggs.

The room remained free of mites for 4 months after which time a low grade infestation was found involving AKR strain mice. Some of these infested animals had been recently imported from the USA. It was concluded therefore that these mice may have been responsible for the reintroduction of mites.

An effort was made to prevent the reintroduction of mites by mice bought from suppliers. It was decided that all mice, except those designated category **** (LAC Accreditation Scheme) or Specified Pathogen Free, would be dipped twice, once on arrival and again 14 days later, and would only be held in rooms on the lower level of the Animal House.

When it was discovered that mites had gained access to the treated rooms, it was felt worthwhile to try dusting with sulphur powder as reported by Madden *et al.* (1954). The first two investigations (experiment 4) successfully eradicated mites. Treated mice appeared healthier and the alopecia associated with infestation regressed. In a large scale trial using the tumbler (Green and Needham, 1974b), two treatments were given which cleared the room of mites. Sulphur had the advantages over the Pyractone product of being easier to use, and eliminating the need to wet the animal.

All mite infested rooms were treated with sulphur which apparently eradicated mites from the Animal House. Unfortunately after 7 months a low grade infestation was found in three rooms. The source was traced to the conventional breeding room which had not been treated or regularly checked in case the breeding schedules were disrupted. In the light of this evidence the breeding room was treated together with all other rooms. This involved treating 25 000 mice and 1000 rats and was carried out easily using the tumbler. Following this treatment no mites were seen for 9 months, when a low grade infestation was discovered in one room. It was then accepted that routine treatments would be carried out at 6-monthly intervals, as complete eradication was probably not possible in such a large colony. This scheme of treatment has now been modified (Needham, 1978).

At the time of writing over 100 000 mice have been treated and only isolated deaths have occurred. Some animals exhibited increased alopecia after treatment and this was investigated. The skin of a mouse that died after treatment with sulphur was examined and basophilic granules were seen in the basal layers of the epithelium (Fig. 18). It was thought possible that these particles were sulphur, which appeared to suggest a sulphur overdose and an experiment was set up to study the effects of an overdose (Cooper and Needham, 1976a).

Experiment 5: A Study of the Effects of the Overapplication of Sulphur to the Skin of Mice

Materials and Methods

Animals

18 adult male and 18 adult female CBA/H-T6Crc mice were issued from the barrier unit and placed six of the same sex to a box.

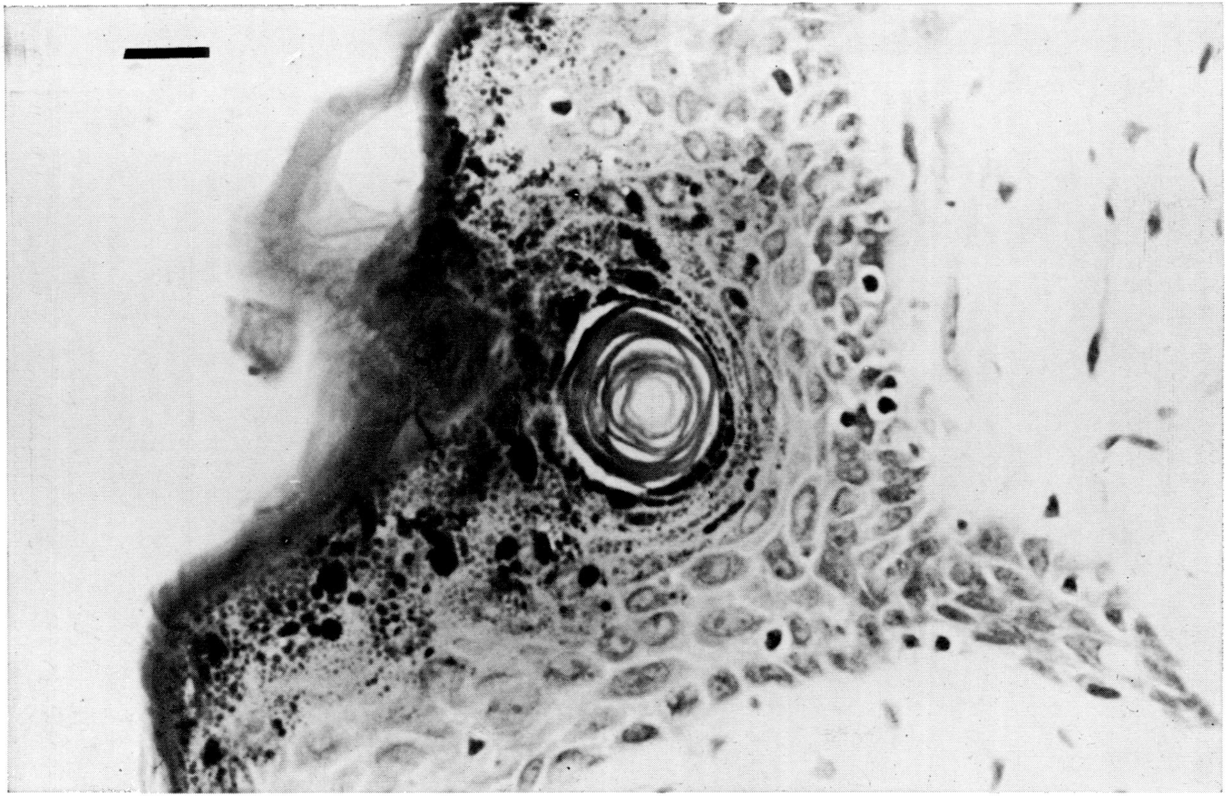

Fig. 18. Mouse skin showing granules in the stratum granulosum. Coles haematoxylin and eosin. Line represents 25 μm.

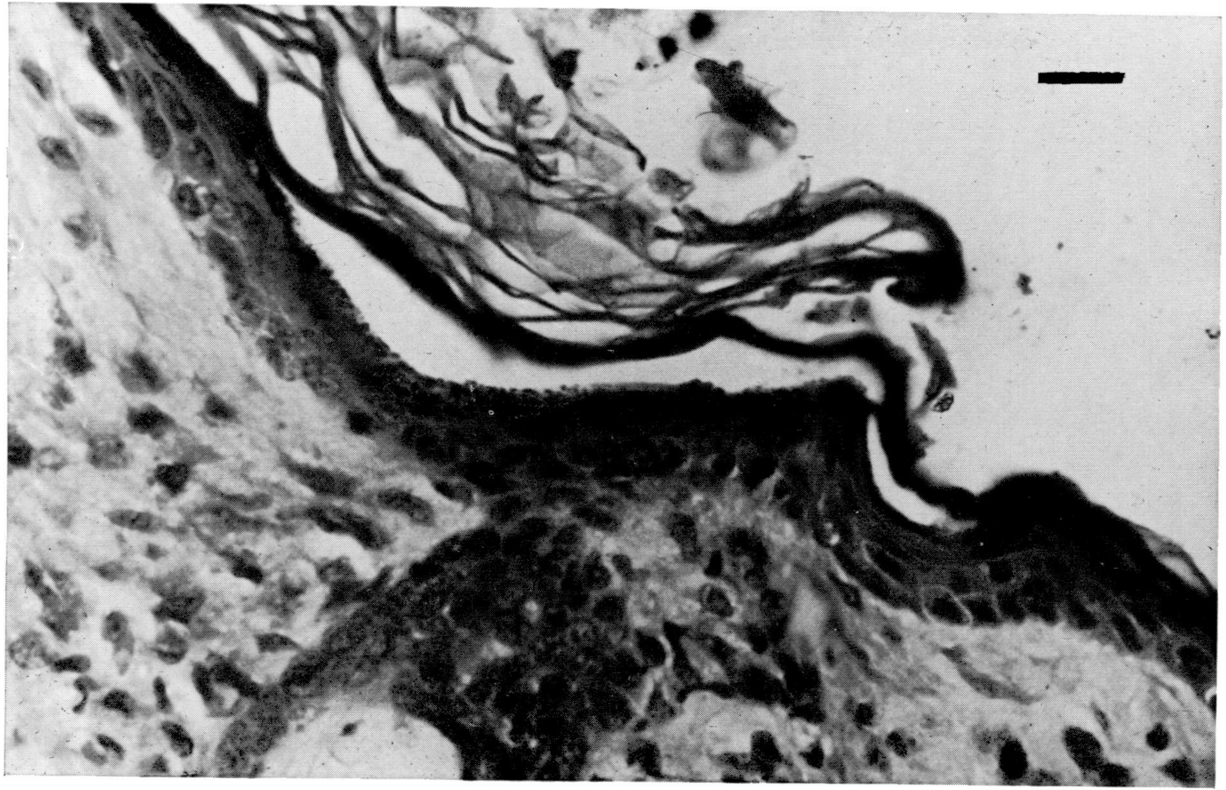

Fig. 19. Mouse skin showing hyperkeratinisation. Coles haematoxylin and eosin. Line represents 25 μm,

Methods

One group of six male mice was treated with sulphur, the chemical being applied by hand and rubbed into the fur of the mice for 3 min. A second group received two treatments 48 h apart and the third control group remained untreated. All mice were killed by intraperitoneal administration of sodium pentobarbitone on day 7 after the initial treatment. A portion of skin was removed from the neck, the back and the right hind leg for histopathological examination. The experiment was repeated with female mice.

Results

108 skin sections were examined and only minor abnormalities were found. All groups of mice, including untreated mice, showed slight hyperkeratinization (excessive accumulation of keratin on the surface of skin) (Fig. 19), and amongst the sulphur rolled groups there were a few cases of parakeratosis (disturbance of the normal architecture of the skin). Only one mouse, that had been rolled twice in sulphur, showed any degree of epithelial thickening. Basophilic granules were observed in the basal layers (stratum granulosum) of the epithelium in sections of skin taken from all groups of mice including control animals (Fig. 18).

The results of this survey were compared with the results obtained from the examination of 20 serial sections of a heavily mite infested CBA mouse. This mouse had not been treated with an acaracide. The skin showed a slight degree of epithelial thickening and patchy hyperkeratinization. Basophilic granules were present in varying numbers, density and distribution. In some sections a mite had been sectioned and was associated with a focus of mononuclear infiltration in the dermis.

Discussion

The study of the effects of a sulphur overdose did not yield conclusive results. Histological examination of a mouse that had died following a routine sulphur treatment showed basophilic granules in the stratum granulosum. These were at first thought to be pathological but granules were later seen in untreated controls as well as treated mice. It was assumed that these were normal and probably associated with the hyperkeratinization.

No difference was seen between the various groups of mice, whether sulphur had been applied once or twice. The cause of the alopecia was not determined but it was thought possible that it may have been due to sulphur occluding the hair follicle and hence contacting the germinating layers at the base of the follicle. A more likely explanation however was that the alopecia seen in the colony was the result of the stress of treatment on debilitated mice.

8

Sub-human Primates

Microbiological Screening

Introduction

The primates are housed in special rooms under strict hygiene control and all staff entering the rooms must wear protective clothing. In one room is the rhesus colony, cynomolgus monkeys in another and marmosets and tamarins in a third. There is only a small yearly turnover (approximately 100) of animals and the majority are involved in long term investigations including transplantation surgery.

The use of large numbers of primates for research purposes has stimulated much work on the microbiology, husbandry and infections of primates (Brown *et al.,* 1973; Deinhardt *et al.,* 1967; Pinkerton, 1968; Ruch, 1959). It has long been known that non-human primates harbour organisms that may be pathogenic to humans, so it is essential that the health of these animals should be carefully observed clinically in order to prevent infections within individual colonies and safeguard personnel from the risk of transmitted infection. Primates used for transplantation studies are regarded as a greater hazard because of their exposure to immunosuppression (van Bekkum, 1970).

It was decided, before monkeys were first introduced into the Animal House, that the health of these animals would be checked by clinical observation, particularly for the first few weeks after arrival of the animal and by microbiological screening of their faeces. The examinations performed were designed to check each animal for the presence of tuberculosis, simian viruses and pathogenic enteric bacteria.

Tuberculosis

Tuberculosis was recognized in primates as long ago as 1892 (Sanyal). This was followed in 1906 when Baermann and Halberstaedter demonstrated an allergic tuberculin reaction in monkeys; White and Fox (1909) used this reaction for the detection of tuberculosis. Schroeder (1938) described the use of the eyelid for this test.

Viruses

Kalter and Heberling (1969) reviewed simian viruses and measures necessary to isolate viruses from primates. *Herpesvirus simiae* (B virus) causes an infection in man with a high mortality rate. The effect on the primate host is to produce mild clinical signs (Keeble, 1968), but in some cases, affected animals may show no clinical signs. The characteristic lesion is an ulcer on the lips, tongue or buccal mucosa (Chaffee, 1972) with a possible transient mucopurulent nasal discharge of up to 10 days duration.

Enteric Organisms

The alimentary tract of primates is colonized by many organisms that may be isolated from human intestines, for example *Escherichia coli* and *Pseudomonas aeruginosa*, and they are also liable to carry *Salmonella* and *Shigella* species with or without clinical signs of illness.

The colonization of primate intestines by these latter two organisms and their effect on the monkey and its contacts has been well documented (Caraway *et al.*, 1968; Cook, 1953a; Lindsey *et al.*, 1971; Rewell and Bridges, 1948; Ruch, 1959). Bach, Fulscher and Harnack (1931) and Carpenter (1968) reported cases of simian to human transmission. It has not been possible to demonstrate the presence of shigellae in wild primates (Carpenter and Cooke, 1965; Takaska *et al.*, 1964) and it is thought that their intestines become colonized by these organisms through initial contacts with humans, when captured and held in compounds. Subsequently the stresses of captivity and transportation may cause symptomless excretors to become clinically ill (Cook, 1969). Whilst sick, the monkeys may infect their primate companions and human contacts if hygienic conditions are not maintained. In one study, it was shown that colonization was unlikely to have occurred in the United Kingdom as exotic strains of *Shigella* species were isolated (Carpenter, 1968).

The pathogenesis of shigella and salmonella infections is very similar. In the terminal stages animals become severely dehydrated, will not eat and usually pass bloody watery faeces. At autopsy, ulceration of the intestinal mucosa is the most common finding. Although there are few recorded cases of transmission of infection from monkeys to man, these organisms present the most constant threat to personnel involved with primates. They may be excreted in the faeces, so regular sampling and examination of stool samples should be carried out.

Table 38

Number of faecal specimens examined from sub-human primates

	Number of samples		
Species	Routine	Disease outbreak	Total
Rhesus	337	267	604
Cynomolgus	405	—	405
Marmosets and tamarins	218	447	665
Baboons	95	—	95
Squirrel	82	32	114
	1137	746	1883

During the period of the investigations recorded here, 1883 samples were examined and Table 38 shows the number of samples obtained from each species. These are recorded under four headings (1) routine sampling, (2) an outbreak of enteritis in rhesus monkeys (*Macaca mulatta*) (Needham, 1975), (3) an outbreak of shigellosis in marmosets (*Callithrix jacchus*) and tamarins (*Saguinus* species) (Cooper and Needham, 1976b) and (4) an outbreak of enteric disease in squirrel monkeys (*Saimiri* species).

Routine Sampling

It was decided that samples would be taken once a month from all cages containing sub-human primates. In addition to the species listed above, samples were examined from cynomolgus monkeys (*Macaca fascicularis*) and baboons (*Papio* species). Faeces samples were also obtained from monkeys observed with diarrhoea.

An Outbreak of Enteritis in Rhesus Monkeys

Diarrhoea was observed on the day following delivery of a batch of 20 female rhesus monkeys. The animals were held in isolation quarters whilst tests were carried out.

An Outbreak of Shigellosis in Marmosets and Tamarins

Prior to the outbreak the majority of the colony had been within the facility for 18 months during which time no clinical illness occurred and they were subjected to the routine tests already detailed. A small additional number of animals were then introduced into the colony and faecal samples were obtained from the entire colony.

After approximately 5 weeks the first signs of clinical illness were observed including the appearance of diarrhoea. The number of clinical cases increased and microbiological tests were carried out including the examination of faecal specimens as well as specimens collected during *post mortem* examinations.

An Outbreak of Enteric Disease in Squirrel Monkeys

Two small groups of squirrel monkeys were held, one group in the infective suite where they were inoculated with a neurotropic virus and a second in the isotope suite. Regular monthly faecal samples were obtained over a period of 1 year until diarrhoea was observed. In view of the long-term nature of the experimental work and the fact that diarrhoea may indicate salmonellosis or shigellosis, it was decided that an attempt must be made to isolate the causal agent. The frequency of faecal sampling was therefore increased but no *post mortem* examinations of dead monkeys were performed.

Tuberculosis

Materials and Method

The examination for tuberculosis is carried out by the veterinary surgeon in the third week after arrival whilst the primate is in isolation (Coid, 1969). The test involves the intrapalpebral injection of 10 000 IU of Mammalian Tuberculin PPD (Ministry of Agriculture, Central Veterinary Laboratory, Weybridge, Surrey). The monkey is then observed for 4 days.

Results

Throughout the 2½-year period covered in this book no cases of monkeys affected by tuberculosis were detected.

Discussion

All new monkeys arriving at this Centre were tuberculin tested for tuberculosis. This involved the testing of approximately 250 monkeys over a period of 2½ years. During this period of time all monkeys tested appeared to be free from infection. This observation would appear to agree with the experience of other workers. Bywater *et al.* (1962) reported an incidence of 1·7% after testing 2301 rhesus monkeys, and Stones (1969) found only five cases during the examination of over 21 000 vervet monkeys (*Cercopithecus aethiops*). Both workers also reported that autopsy diagnosis of tuberculosis did not correlate with the tuberculin test results. At this Centre, autopsies were not performed on monkeys unless the procedure was essential to an experiment. During one such autopsy, lung nodules were found suggestive of tuberculosis, but culture did not yield any organisms.

In view of the failure to culture organisms from the lung nodules and the reported lack of correlation between tuberculin tests and autopsy findings, other methods of diagnosis were considered. Thoracic X-ray examinations could be carried out and it was known that one supplier used this in conjunction with the tuberculin test. However, this was not adopted as it was felt that the time involved sedating and transporting the monkeys was not justified. Furthermore the test would have necessitated the removal of the monkey from the isolation room into the Animal House before its isolation period was over. A more feasible procedure was to increase the frequency of tuberculin testing so that each animal was tested at least twice whilst in isolation.

Viruses

Method

No laboratory investigations were undertaken to examine monkeys for the presence of viruses. A visual inspection of the buccal mucosa was made by the veterinary surgeon, when monkeys were sedated for tuberculin testing.

Results

Two monkeys were killed when small blisters were found on the buccal mucosa. No confirmatory investigations for example serology, were undertaken.

Discussion

Virologically, the examination of the monkeys was limited to visual inspection of the buccal mucosa. During the $2\frac{1}{2}$-year period, no obvious cases of infection occurred. Four monkeys exhibited lesions and all were killed with the exception of two: one of these was sent to the Microbiological Research Establishment at Porton and was subsequently shown to be free from infection, and the second exhibited a lesion that was obviously the result of trauma. The presence of lesions around the mouth may be due to a host of causal agents, but it was felt that the difficulties of a positive diagnosis were such that it was safer to kill the monkey rather than risk a serious infection in personnel.

Enteric Organisms: Routine Sampling of Faeces

Materials and Methods

Faeces were obtained from the tray under each cage (Fig. 20). A visual inspection of the tray contents was made and a fresh sample of faeces selected (Needham, 1977), and collected using a spoon contained in a universal bottle (Sterilin Ltd, Teddington, Middlesex).

Samples of faeces were collected monthly from all monkeys not in isolation quarters. Animals in isolation were sampled on the first 3 days after delivery and again after 4 weeks. The bottles of faeces were dipped

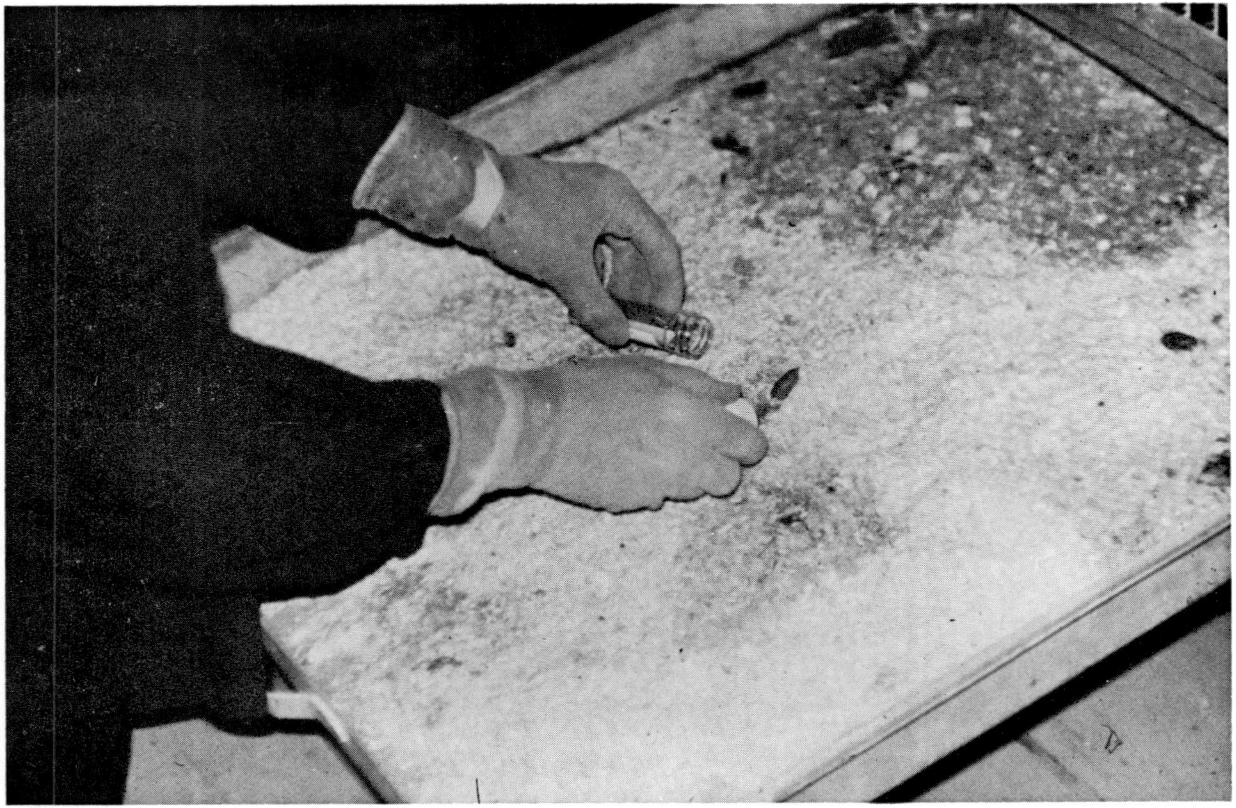

Fig. 20. Collection of monkey faeces from the undercage tray.

in 5% chloros and then placed in a plastic bag which was sealed and dipped before being placed in a second plastic bag which was similarly treated before transport to the laboratory. The faeces were then inoculated on to deoxycholate citrate agar and in to selenite F medium.

Results

A total of 1137 samples of faeces was examined (Table 38). Six isolates of *Shigella sonnei* were obtained from 337 samples of rhesus monkey faeces and one isolate of *Shigella dysenteriae* from 405 samples of cynomolgus monkey faeces. Baboons, squirrel monkeys and marmosets did not yield shigellae or salmonellae.

An Outbreak of Enteritis in Rhesus Monkeys

Materials and Methods

Animals

Twenty female rhesus monkeys, weighing 4·5 kg were delivered from a commercial supplier in the late afternoon and were immediately housed in an isolation (quarantine) room. They were given water and feeding was commenced next day.

Antibiotics Used

(a) Colistin Methane Sulphonate, "Colomycin", Pharmax Ltd, Crayford, Kent.
(b) Chloramphenicol, "Intramycetin", Parke Davis & Co., Hounslow, Middx.
(c) Ampicillin, "Penbritin", Beecham Veterinary Products, Manor Royal, Crawley, Sussex.
(d) Oxytetracycline, "Terramycin", Pfizer Ltd, Sandwich, Kent.

Also administered was iron "Imferon", Fisons Ltd, Loughborough, Leicestershire and 4·3% dextrose in 0·18% saline, Travenol Ltd (Baxters), Thetford, Norfolk. See Table 39 for treatment regimes.

Table 39

Treatment regimes for rhesus monkeys in isolation

Time post delivery	Monkey number	Agent	Dose per day	Duration in days
1 day	19, 20	Colistin	250 000 units intra-muscular	5
4 days	7, 8	Colistin	250 000 units intra-muscular	5
7 weeks	7, 8	Chloram-phenicol	75 mg intra-muscular	5
4 days	15, 16	Colistin	250 000 units intra-muscular	5
$8\frac{1}{2}$ weeks	15, 16	Chloram-phenicol	75 mg intra-muscular	5
		Oxytetra-cycline	1 mg/ml in drinking water	5
		Dextrose saline	150 ml subcutaneously	8
7 weeks	5, 6	Ampicillin	75 mg intra-muscular	4
		Imferon	50 mg intra-muscular	4
$7\frac{1}{2}$ weeks	5, 6	Oxytetra-cycline	1 mg/ml in drinking water	5
$9\frac{1}{2}$ weeks	1	Chloram-phenicol	75 mg intra-muscular	3

Methods

Clinical Observations

The morning after delivery, blood stained faeces were found on the tray under one cage. Three days later the monkeys in another two cages were passing bloody faeces. After a further 7 weeks, diarrhoea consisting mainly of watery faeces with blood and mucus, was found on the tray under two cages. The two monkeys in one cage had passed blood-stained stools previously in the outbreak and one was clinically sick. Finally, at 9 weeks post delivery, the monkeys in two more cages were involved, and all were showing signs of clinical illness. Two monkeys, which were housed together, had a previous history of diarrhoea.

Microbiology

A total of 267 samples of faeces was examined. The samples were obtained twice weekly from all monkeys as well as from cases of clinical illness.

The faeces were plated out on to deoxycholate citrate agar (DCA) and into selenite F and any non-lactose fermenting colonies were screened for *Salmonella* and *Shigella* species. Any suspect colonies were subjected to biochemical tests and results were confirmed by serological tests if indicated.

Following the initial outbreak of diarrhoea, 88 isolates of commensal intestinal flora were studied from this batch of rhesus monkeys and a fresh batch subsequently delivered to the isolation room. Isolates were obtained from DCA plates and antibiotic sensitivity tests were performed on diagnostic sensitivity test agar with the addition of 7·5% lysed blood using "Multodisks" (Oxoid Ltd, Basingstoke, Hants.).

Results

Whilst in isolation five monkeys died out of nine observed to be suffering with diarrhoea. Four isolates of *Shigella* species were obtained from the 267 specimens of faeces examined, which represents a 1·5% recovery rate (Table 40).

Table 40

Shigella isolation from rhesus monkeys

Monkey number	Time post delivery	Isolate
19, 20	1 day	*Shigella sonnei*
5, 6	7 weeks	*Shigella flexneri* 2
5, 6	7·5 weeks	*Shigella flexneri* 2
7, 8	7 weeks	*Shigella flexneri* Y

The outbreak of disease was noted to occur in two distinct phases. The first began on the day after delivery and lasted for approximately 10 days and the second occurred 7 weeks after delivery and lasted for 17 days. It was observed that when diarrhoea was present at these two periods of time there was an increase in the isolation rate of commensal organisms including *Pseudomonas* species, *Providence* groups and *Escherichia coli.*

Between weeks 2 and 7 after delivery of the monkeys, the number of commensal organisms isolated was reduced and this coincided with the absence of diarrhoea. The antibiotics used during the initial outbreak of diarrhoea were not successful in preventing the recurrence of diarrhoea at 7 weeks (Table 41). Numerous isolates of commensal organisms were

Table 41

Results of treatments to rhesus monkeys

Monkey number	Antibiotic	Time post delivery	Result
19, 20	Colistin methane sulphonate	1 day	Survived
7, 8	Colistin methane sulphonate	4 days	Survived
7, 8	Chloramphenicol	7 weeks	No. 7 died after 2 days. No. 8 survived
15, 16	Colistin methane sulphonate	4 days	Survived
15, 16	Chloramphenicol Oxytetracycline	8·5 weeks	Both died after 8 days
5, 6	Ampicillin	7 weeks	No. 5 died after 4 days. No. 6 survived
6	Oxytetracycline	7·5 weeks	Survived
1	Chloramphenicol	9 weeks	Died after 3 days

Table 42

Number of commensal organisms isolated from 88 samples of faeces from healthy rhesus monkeys tested for antibiotic sensitivity

Organism	Number of isolates
Proteus spp.	24
Proteus vulgaris	7
Proteus mirabilis	5
Proteus morganii	1
Proteus rettgeri	2
Escherichia coli	22
Citrobacter sp.	6
Pseudomonas spp.	7
Enterobacter sp.	14

Table 43

Antibiotic sensitivity of commensal organisms from healthy rhesus monkeys

Organism	Antibiotic and percentage of isolates sensitive																	
	Tetracycline	Chloramphenicol	Cephaloridine	Erythromycin	Kanamycin	Penicillin	Ampicillin	Streptomycin	Tylosin	Chlortetracycline	Colistin methane sulphonate	Furazolidone	Neomycin	Oxytetracycline	Methicillin	Sulfamethoxazole/ Trimethoprim[a]	Carbenicillin
Proteus spp.	8·3	8·3	0	0	41·7	0	0	20·8	0	4·2	8·3	4·2	62·5	8·3	0	29·2	54·2
P. vulgaris	0	5·7	0	0	71·4	0	0	57·1	0	0	14·3	0	83·7	0	0	28·6	14·3
P. mirabilis	0	0	0	0	40·0	0	60·0	40·0	0	0	0	0	20·0	0	40·0	40·0	40·0
P. morganii	0	0	0	0	100	0	0	100	0	0	0	0	100	0	100	100	100
P. rettgeri	50·0	0	0	0	50·0	0	0	50·0	0	50·0	50·0	0	100	50·0	0	0	NT
E. coli	22·7	40·7	18·2	0	27·3	0	0	40·9	0	13·6	50·0	45·6	81·8	9·1	4·5	59·1	36·4
Citrobacter spp.	33·3	16·7	0	0	33·3	0	0	0	0	0	0	33·3	100	0	0	50·0	33·3
Pseudomonas spp.	0	0	0	0	0	0	0	14·3	0	0	0	0	42·9	0	0	0	14·3
Enterobacter sp.	28·3	7·1	7·1	0	71·4	0	0	28·5	0	14·3	50·0	35·7	92·9	21·4	0	28·5	14·3

[a] Septrin; NT, Not tested.

obtained from the survey of faeces from healthy monkeys (Table 42) and the sensitivity of these to antibiotics is shown in Table 43.

Since the transfer of the remaining unaffected monkeys to the main colony, no cases of diarrhoea have been observed and only small numbers of commensal organisms have been isolated.

Shigellosis Outbreak in Marmosets and Tamarins

Materials and Methods

Materials

Antibiotic Used

"Neobiotic P" (Neomycin with Pamine, Upjohn Ltd, Fleming Way, Crawley, Sussex).

Methods

During the outbreak, 447 samples of faeces were examined. These may be divided into those obtained during the 6-week acute phase of the outbreak and those obtained in the 8-week period after the final antibiotic treatment of the colony.

Acute Phase

Every monkey that died during this period was examined *post mortem*. A sample of faeces was obtained from the caecum and plated on to deoxycholate citrate agar and into selenite F. Antibiotic sensitivity tests were performed on any isolates of pathogenic enteric organisms. A careful examination was made of all organs at autopsy and specimens collected for histological preparation. All examinations were performed in an exhaust ventilated safety cabinet (Microflow Ltd, Fleet, Hampshire). Table 44 summarizes the chronological order of deaths during this phase.

Two weeks after the appearance of diarrhoea, faecal samples were obtained from every cage, once weekly for 3 weeks. All isolates of *Shigella sonnei* and commensal enteric organisms were tested for sensitivity to antibiotics.

Table 44

Summary of deaths of animals during the Shigellosis outbreak

Monkey	Days after start of outbreak
Marmoset (adult)	16
Marmoset (young)	18
Marmoset (adult)	20
Marmoset (adult)	23
Marmoset (adult)	25
Tamarin (baby)	27
Marmoset (adult)	27
3 Marmosets (adult)	29
2 Marmosets (baby)	32
Marmoset (adult)	32
Marmoset (adult)	35
Marmoset (adult)	38

After Treatment

Three weeks after the first death occurred, the entire colony was treated with antibiotic. Six millilitres of Neobiotic P was added to 310 ml of drinking water which was renewed daily for 10 days, the average consumption being 15 ml of water per monkey per day.

It was decided to check the colony for the presence of symptomless excretors of *Shigella sonnei* and to determine whether the commensal enteric organisms had developed resistance to neomycin. Samples of faeces were obtained as before from every cage on three consecutive days commencing at days 7, 14, 42, 49 and 56 after the final treatment. All isolates of *Shigella, Salmonella* and commensal enteric organisms were subjected to antibiotic sensitivity testing.

Results

During the outbreak 15 monkeys died. A total of 447 faecal samples was examined, 172 in the acute phase and 275 in the chronic phase; 11 isolates of *Shigella sonnei* were obtained during the acute phase and four isolates of this organism and one isolate of *Salmonella irumu* were obtained during the chronic phase.

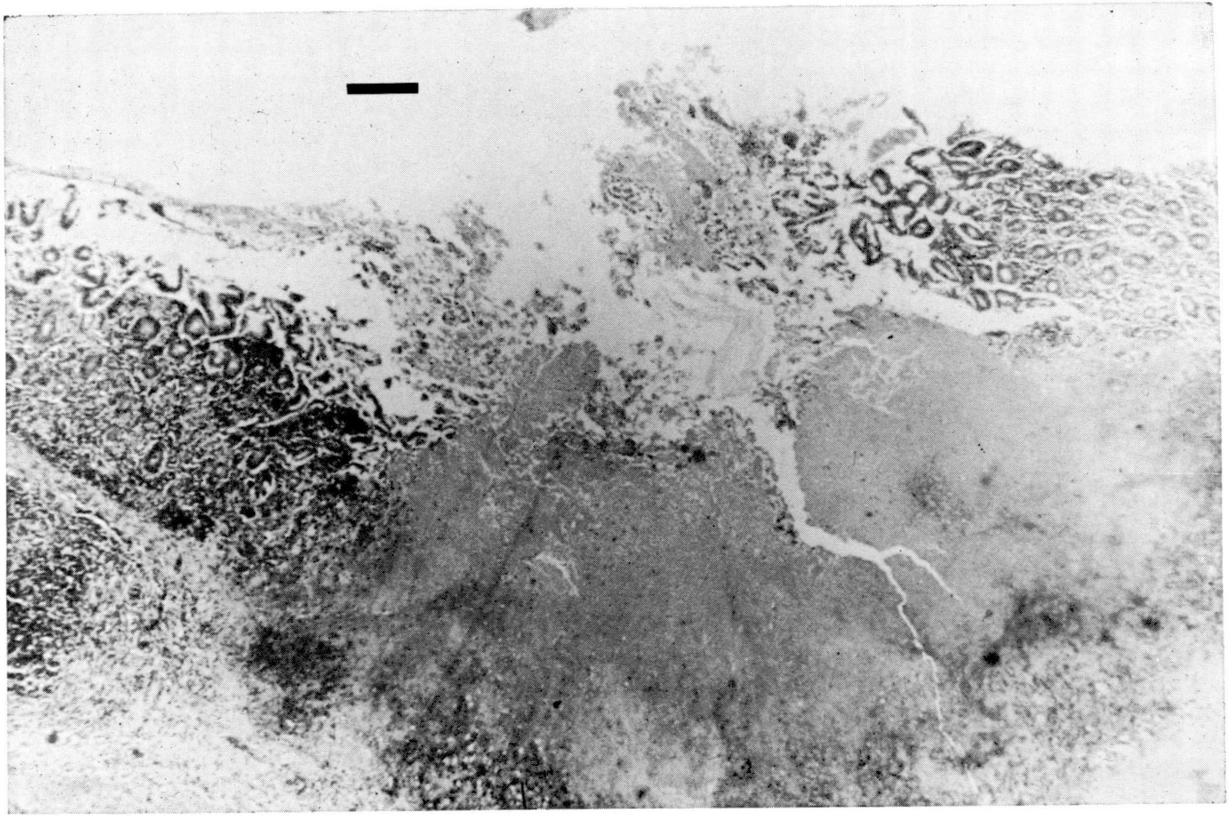

Fig. 21. Caecum of marmoset infected with *Shigella sonnei* showing an ulcer with debris and associated haemorrhage. Coles haematoxylin and eosin. Line represents 500 μm.

At the commencement of the outbreak the only organism isolated from faeces was *Pseudomonas aeruginosa* which was thought responsible for the diarrhoea. This possibility was reinforced when this organism was cultured from the caeca of the first four monkeys to die.

Three weeks after the initial case of diarrhoea, faeces were obtained from all cages and four isolates of *Shigella sonnei* were obtained. This was followed by the isolation 1 day later of *Shigella sonnei* from the caecal contents of a dead marmoset.

The monkeys all presented similar clinico-pathological signs. Affected animals were dehydrated and the anal region was soiled with dried blood and faeces. Internally, the caecum was ulcerated and contained free blood mixed with fluid faeces. In a few cases the ulceration was found extending into the large intestine. No faeces of normal consistency were seen. Both the caecal and mesenteric lymph nodes were enlarged. The mesenteric blood vessels were dilated to varying degrees.

Histological examination showed erosions of the mucosa of the large intestine, which had in some cases progressed to ulceration (Fig. 21). There were haemorrhages on the periphery of the ulcers and their floor

Table 45

Number of commensal organisms tested for antibiotic sensitivity following isolation from marmosets and tamarins faecal samples

Organism	Number of isolates examined during 0–14 days after final antibiotic treatment of colony
Escherichia coli	48
Aeromonas sp.	11
Pseudomonas spp.	4
Proteus spp.	6
Citrobacter sp.	2
	Number of isolates examined during 42–56 days after final antibiotic treatment of colony
Escherichia coli	14
Aeromonas sp.	2
Pseudomonas spp.	4
Proteus spp.	5
Enterobacter sp.	2

was composed of cellular debris. The sub-mucosa usually showed a cellular response composed of neutrophils and mononuclear cells.

Large numbers of commensal organisms were isolated with *Escherichia coli* being isolated most frequently (Table 45). It was found that the sensitivity of the commensal organisms to neomycin decreased in the first 2 weeks following the final treatment of the colony (Table 46), but this resistance decreased over the following weeks (Table 47). It was also observed that the isolates of *Shigella sonnei* following treatment were less sensitive to neomycin (Table 49). Furthermore the administration of this antibiotic did not prevent deaths occurring (Table 48).

Repeated sampling of faeces revealed the presence of symptomless excretors.

Table 46

Antibiotic sensitivity of commensal organisms isolated 0–14 days after final treatment of the colony

Antibiotic	Organism and percentage sensitivity				
	Escherichia coli	*Aeromonas* sp.	*Pseudomonas* spp.	*Proteus* spp.	*Citrobacter* sp.
Tetracycline	24	29	0	0	50
Chloramphenicol	52	46	0	33	100
Cephaloridine	32	9	0	17	0
Erythromycin	0	0	0	0	0
Kanamycin	0	9	0	0	0
Penicillin	0	0	0	0	0
Ampicillin	0	0	0	0	0
Streptomycin	14	0	0	0	0
Tylosin	0	0	0	0	0
Chlortetracycline	10	9	0	0	0
Colistin methane sulphonate	96	100	100	17	100
Furazolidone	92	37	0	0	100
Neomycin	0	9	0	33	0
Oxytetracycline	18	18	0	0	50
Methicillin	0	0	0	0	0
Sulfamethoxazole-Trimethoprim (Septrin)	86	54	0	50	100
Carbenicillin	26	0	75	66	0
Gentamicin	90	100	100	83	100

Table 47

Antibiotic sensitivity of commensal organisms isolated 42–56 days after final treatment of the colony

Antibiotic	Organism and percentage sensitivity				
	Escherichia coli	*Aeromonas* sp.	*Pseudomonas* spp.	*Proteus* spp.	*Enterobacter* sp.
Tetracycline	14	50	0	20	0
Chloramphenicol	86	50	0	40	0
Cephaloridine	66	0	0	40	0
Erythromycin	0	0	0	0	0
Kanamycin	28	0	0	40	100
Penicillin	0	0	0	0	0
Ampicillin	0	0	0	0	0
Streptomycin	30	0	0	20	0
Tylosin	0	0	0	0	0
Chlortetracycline	0	0	0	20	0
Colistin methane sulphonate	92	50	100	60	100
Furazolidone	92	50	0	0	0
Neomycin	28	0	0	80	100
Oxytetracycline	28	0	0	40	0
Methicillin	0	0	0	0	0
Sulfamethoxazole-Trimethoprim (Septrin)	51	0	0	40	0
Carbenicillin	86	0	75	80	0
Gentamicin	100	100	100	100	100

Table 48

Results of treatments of marmosets

Number of marmosets	Number of days after start of outbreak	Duration of treatment in days	Result
2	18	6	Survived
2	19	6	1 died
1	24	1	Died
Entire colony	29	10	3 died after 3 days 1 died after 6 days 1 died after 9 days

Table 49

Antibiotic sensitivity of *Shigella sonnei* and *Salmonella irumu* isolated from marmosets and tamarins

Organism examined	Number of isolates examined	Antibiotic and percentage sensitivity																
		Tetracycline	Chloramphenicol	Cephaloridine	Erythromycin	Kanamycin	Penicillin	Ampicillin	Streptomycin	Tylosin	Chlortetracycline	Colistin methane sulphonate	Furazolidone	Neomycin	Oxytetracycline	Sulfamethoxazole-Trimethoprim (Septrin)	Carbenicillin	Gentamicin
S. sonnei isolated during first 6 weeks of outbreak	11	0	92	72	0	46	0	0	9	0	0	46	92	92	0	36	81	100
S. sonnei isolated during 42–56 days after final antibiotic treatment of colony	8	0	77	77	0	44	0	0	0	0	0	77	77	55	0	66	88	88
Salmonella irumu isolated during 42–56 days after final antibiotic treatment of colony	3	33	100	100	0	66	0	0	66	0	0	100	0	100	0	66	66	100

Outbreaks of Enteric Disease in Squirrel Monkeys

Materials and Methods

Materials

Animals

The monkeys involved were adult females in two groups, one group of 11 held in the infected suite, a second group of six held in the isotope suite. Prior to the outbreak they had been held in the suites for 1 year.

Antibiotics used

(a) Oxytetracycline, "Terramycin", Pfizer Ltd, Sandwich, Kent.
(b) Chlortetracycline, "Aureomycin", Cyanamid of Great Britain Ltd, Fareham Road, Gosport, Hants.
(c) Furaltadone, "Furasol", Smith Kline and French Laboratories Ltd, Welwyn Garden City, Herts.

Glucose was also administered. See Table 50 for treatment regimes.

Table 50
Treatment regimes for squirrel monkeys

Time after start of outbreak in days	Source	Agent	Dose per day in drinking water	Duration in days
16	Isotope suite	Aureomycin	0·1 mg/ml	5
		Glucose	1 teaspoon/ 250 ml	5
21	Isotope suite	Terramycin	1 mg/ml	4
25	Isotope suite	Aureomycin	0·1 mg/ml	5
30	Isotope suite	Furasol	20 mg/ml	19
17	Infective suite	Aureomycin	0·1 mg/ml	5
		Glucose	1 teaspoon/ 250 ml	5

Methods

Clinical Observations

Diarrhoea was first observed in the isotope suite and a sample of faeces was obtained from the tray under each cage. Four days later, diarrhoea was found in monkeys in the infected suite and faeces were obtained. One monkey in this suite died, followed by a second 9 days later. As diarrhoea was persisting, faeces were again collected and antibiotic treatment was commenced (Table 50). Whilst antibiotics were being administered further deaths occurred in both suites although no pattern of deaths was noticed amongst control and experimental groups. Tables 51 and 52 summarize the chronological order of deaths in both suites.

Microbiology

Samples of faeces were obtained monthly from both groups of monkeys until diarrhoea was seen in the isotope suite when they were collected as recorded in Tables 51 and 52.

Throughout the outbreak the faeces were only taken from the trays

Table 51

Summary of observations and results of treatments to squirrel monkeys held in infected suite

Time after start of outbreak in days	Faecal sample	Treatment given	Result
0	Yes	None	Nothing abnormal
6	Yes—diarrhoea	None	Monkey 11 died
15	No	None	Monkey 5 died
17	Yes—diarrhoea	Aureomycin	No change
23	Yes—diarrhoea	None	Monkey 7 died
24	No	None	Monkeys 2 and 4 died
28	No	None	Monkeys 3 and 6 died
29	No	None	Monkeys 9 and 10 died
31	No	None	Monkey 7 died
33	No	None	Monkey 8 died

Table 52

Summary of observations and results of treatments to squirrel monkeys held in isotope suite

Time after start of outbreak in days	Faecal sample	Treatment given	Result
0	Yes	None	Nothing abnormal
2	Yes—diarrhoea	None	Nothing abnormal
16	Yes—diarrhoea	Aureomycin	No change
21	No	Terramycin	No change
25	No	Aureomycin	No change
30	No	Furasol	No change
33	Yes—diarrhoea	Furasol	No change
39	No	Furasol	1 monkey died
43	No	Furasol	1 monkey died
45	No	Furasol	1 monkey died
47	No	Furasol	Remaining 3 monkeys sent to M.R.E.

MRE, Microbiological Research Establishment, Porton.

under the cages and were inoculated into selenite F and on to deoxycholate citrate agar. No antibiotic sensitivity tests or *post mortem* examinations were performed.

Results

The outbreaks of disease resulted in the death of all 11 monkeys in the infected suite and three out of the six monkeys in the isotope suite. At no time was any enteric pathogen isolated from faecal material, and only small numbers of commensal organisms were obtained.

Discussion

A great amount of data was obtained from the sampling of monkey faeces for enteric organisms. A total of 1883 faecal samples was examined over a $2\frac{1}{2}$-year period. Only seven isolates of *Shigella* species were obtained from the routine testing of 1137 samples of faeces, representing a recovery rate of 0·6%. Of these, six isolates of *Shigella sonnei* were obtained from 337 samples of faeces from rhesus monkeys and one isolate of *Shigella dysenteriae* from 405 samples from cynomolgus monkeys. None of these animals showed clinical signs of illness. This isolation rate is extremely low when compared to other workers. Weil *et al.* (1971) reported an incidence of 67·5% of *Shigella* species from a batch of 40 rhesus monkeys. The apparent absence of colonization by *Shigella* may have been due to several factors. As it was thought possible that failure to detect shigellae may have been due to unsuitable media, stock strains of shigellae and salmonella were deliberately inoculated into animal faeces which were then included with uninoculated faeces and plated on to deoxycholate citrate agar and into selenite F. A coding system was used, so that the member of staff handling the specimens could not differentiate inoculated faeces from uninoculated. Both test organisms were successfully recovered so it was concluded that the media used and the faecal screening technique was efficient.

When an isolate of *Shigella* species was found, it was tested for sensitivity to antibiotics. All isolates were sensitive to colistin methane sulphonate (Table 53) and this was used for treatment of the condition: it was administered by intra-muscular injection at a dose of 75 mg/monkey/day for five consecutive days. This antibiotic was chosen in preference to sulfamethoxazole/trimethoprim (Septrin) as Lexomboon *et al.* (1972) had demonstrated 100% sensitivity to colistin with shigellae isolated from children; 7 days after the withdrawal of treatment, samples of faeces were obtained on three consecutive days. In all seven cases no

Table 53

Sensitivity of *Shigella sonnei* isolates obtained from routine faecal samples of monkeys

Antibiotic	Number of isolates sensitive
Streptomycin	4/5
Colistin methane sulphonate	5/5
Sulfamethoxazole-Trimethoprim (Septrin)	5/5
Sulfamethoxazole	4/5
Trimethoprim	4/5

isolates of *Shigella* species were obtained, and hence it was concluded that the monkeys concerned were free from infection.

It may be argued that routine sampling of monkey faeces is not worthwhile considering the time and expense involved when there appears to be a very low incidence of infection. Caraway *et al.* (1968), having found a similarly low incidence (3%) stated that the USAF School of Aerospace Medicine terminated the routine screening of monkeys. However, it must be considered that the object of screening is to protect the remainder of the colony and also personnel. It was felt that this objective over-ruled the low incidence and that negative results were valuable as background data for future reference.

In order that incoming batches of monkeys were screened as thoroughly and quickly as possible, a policy was instituted whereby newly delivered monkeys in isolation were faecal sampled for the first 3 days at the Centre. This procedure was of value when one particular batch of new rhesus monkeys were found with diarroea.

The outbreak of disease occurred in two distinct phases, the first phase lasting 10 days commencing 1 day after delivery and the second lasting for $2\frac{1}{2}$ weeks commencing 7 weeks after delivery. The initial outbreak of diarrhoea was not adequately controlled and this may have been due to one or more factors. In some instances, principally at weekends, faeces were obtained up to 48 h after the onset of diarrhoea; where this occurred, care was taken to select the freshest faeces on the undercage tray. It was also the practice to administer antibiotics to clinical cases as soon as diarrhoea was noticed as this had been apparently effective in dealing with the first seven cases of *Shigella* infection. In some instances, antibiotic treatment was commenced before a faecal sample was obtained and it was felt that organisms may have been suppressed.

In the first outbreak of enteritis, colistin methane sulphonate was administered because of its previous successful use. However, this antibiotic did not prevent a recurrence of disease, as the treated monkeys were observed to be suffering from diarrhoea in the second phase (Table 39), 5 weeks later. It is possible that this was due to too short a period of treatment, or alternatively that the monkeys were reinfected.

When the second phase of enteritis occurred it was decided that treatment had to be attempted using other antibiotics. From the literature there appeared to be a considerable difference of opinion as to the most suitable treatment (Lindsey *et al.*, 1971; Cooke, 1969; Arya *et al.*, 1973). Ampicillin was reported to have been successfully used for the treatment of human shigellosis (Haltalin *et al.*, 1972). It was decided, however, to use chloramphenicol, oxytetracycline and ampicillin but their use did not prevent the deaths of five monkeys (Table 41); oral and parental methods of administration were used but neither method proved successful.

The clinical onset of disease was rapid. Animals with diarrhoea would appear slightly unwell but could within 24 h present signs of severe illness including blood stained faeces, and death usually followed quickly. The rapid development of clinical illness meant that, in some cases, treatment was initiated too late.

Throughout the outbreak, no definite evidence was obtained as to the cause of the diarrhoea although *Shigella* species were isolated on four occasions involving animals in three separate cages. It was finally concluded that the outbreak may have been caused by *Shigella* species which were not detected in routine sampling of newly imported monkeys or by overgrowth of one or more normally commensal enteric organisms perhaps combined with the carriage of *Shigella* species.

If the outbreak was due to *Shigella,* why was it not possible to isolate the organism? It has already been stated in the results that large numbers of enteric commensal organisms were isolated during the two episodes of diarrhoea. These may have caused the failure to isolate *Shigella* species more frequently. Work performed by Hentges (1967) showed that *Shigella flexneri* was inhibited by *Klebsiella* species and Stokes (1973) reported a degree of inhibition by *Proteus* and *Pseudomonas* species. Another factor already mentioned was the administration of antibiotics prior to faeces sampling. It is also possible that more shigella may have been isolated if autopsies had been carried out and caecal material examined as this would have yielded more reliable results than faeces obtained from the undercage tray.

It would be expected that in cases of enteritis the number of commensal organisms in the faeces would be reduced due to the dilution effect of the increased fluid content and also the accelerated movement of the contents in the intestine. However, the increased isolation rate of normal commensal organisms during the outbreak suggested that these organisms were behaving as pathogens. It was not possible to establish whether these organisms were the sole cause of diarrhoea or secondary invaders following an initial shigella infection. Literature available on the role of commensals in enteritis is scanty, although commensal enteric organisms may cause disease outbreaks. It is well known that enteropathogenic *Escherichia coli* causes disease in human infants (South, 1971) and can be isolated from the faeces of laboratory animals (Schiff *et al.*, 1972). Arya *et al.* (1973) made reference to *Arizona* species and *Providence* groups causing deaths in rhesus monkeys and Rewell and Bridges (1948) suggested that *Proteus morganii* was responsible for ulceration and inflammation of the intestines of primates. Thus it is obvious that more work must be performed to study the role of commensals in enteritis.

After the second phase of the outbreak, a study was initiated in healthy rhesus monkeys already released from the isolation quarters, examining all species of enteric organisms isolated from the routine sampling of faeces on deoxycholate citrate agar plates and testing the isolates for sensitivity to antibiotics. The results of this study are displayed in Table 43.

From this small study it was apparent that there was no antibiotic to which all isolates were sensitive, but neomycin had the widest spectrum of activity. It was also observed that normally only one species of organism was isolated, and mixed cultures were unusual.

Two months after the last case of enteritis, the remaining 15 monkeys were transferred from the isolation quarters to the main colony. Repeated sampling of faeces has only revealed small numbers of commensals and the monkeys have remained healthy. Four further batches of rhesus monkeys have been screened on arrival at this Centre and results have confirmed those shown in Table 43. In several cases the organisms isolated have been resistant to all antibiotics involved in the test and this is probably acquired when the monkeys are exposed to antibiotics at the importer's premises. The use of antibiotics by suppliers is widespread and they appear to be used without thought of the consequences. One supplier presented a health certificate with a list of antibiotics which had been administered to treat cases of enteritis including seven different agents. This indiscriminate use of antibiotics can cause complications in subsequent treatment whilst the primate is involved in experiments and is of very doubtful clinical value anyway.

A decision must be made when diarrhoea is first observed, as to the best action to take. It is essential that a faecal specimen is first obtained for microbiological examination; there are then several possible courses of action. If the monkey appears to have no chance of survival as assessed by the veterinary surgeon in charge of the case, then it is probably desirable to kill the animal immediately and hope that the causal agent will not be transmitted to the rest of the colony. If treatment is indicated then the monkey should, if possible, be removed from the colony and housed separately in order to minimize the spread of a possible infection. Unfortunately, at this Centre space limitations do not permit this course of action, but wherever possible affected monkeys are moved away from unaffected animals.

Treatment of affected animals is not without hazards. Antibiotics may prevent the isolation of the causative organism, induce resistance in enteric organisms and may prolong the outbreak (Aserkoff and Bennett, 1969; Dixon, 1965) although, as recorded by Jafary and Burke (1970), this is an acceptable risk in long term cases of infection.

By far the most serious case of disease was an outbreak of shigellosis in the marmoset and tamarin colony. During the acute phase 15 animals died and many more were affected. Occasionally isolates of *Shigella sonnei* are still being obtained. Some of the conclusions reached from experience gained earlier with rhesus monkeys were applied to this outbreak. It was decided that autopsies should be carried out as the animals were being used in experiments and their small size permitted them to be autopsied within a safety hood.

Throughout the outbreak the emphasis was placed on hygienic precautions, particularly before laboratory diagnosis was completed. These precautions included the posting of warning notices, the limiting of entry to one member of staff, the movement of cages so that all infected cages were grouped together, provision of a formalin footbath inside the door and wiping the floors, walls and door handles with formalin daily. Whenever possible, the technician responsible for the room only entered once a day. Hygienic precautions were extended to the laboratory. Carcasses were transported in two plastic bags, both of which had been dipped in 5% chloros. The animal's body was placed inside an exhaust ventilated safety cabinet, and personnel wore gowns, masks, gloves and a hat whilst examining the carcass. At the end of a *post mortem* examination the body was placed in two plastic bags prior to incineration, instruments were soaked for 1 h in chloros and then boiled and all surfaces were cleaned with chloros. It was felt that these stringent precautions would adequately protect personnel whilst allowing *post mortem* examinations to be carried out.

The course of this outbreak was similar in some ways to the outbreak in rhesus monkeys. The first cases of enteritis yielded *Pseudomonas aeruginosa* and it was thought that this organism was responsible for the outbreak. This appeared to be confirmed by the isolation of this organism from the first four autopsies.

After 3 weeks the incidence of clinical symptoms increased and faeces were obtained from all cages for bacteriological examination. This yielded four isolates of *Shigella sonnei*. As a precaution these isolates were subjected to antibiotic sensitivity testing. Next day a marmoset died and *Shigella sonnei* was isolated from caecal contents. As the outbreak progressed, further isolates were obtained from caecal contents at autopsy and classical pathological lesions of shigellosis were seen.

Antibiotic treatment was not commenced until 4 weeks after the start of the outbreak. It had been decided to withhold treatment as long as possible because the isolates of *Pseudomonas aeruginosa* were very resistant to antibiotics and also there was the danger of development of resistance in other groups of bacteria. Further, the most suitable antibiotic was gentamicin, but this could not be used in the Animal House as it was the drug used at the adjoining Northwick Park Hospital for pseudomonas infections and as a precaution its use was prohibited. When treatment was commenced, the antibiotic used was neomycin. This was chosen based on the sensitivity tests of the *Shigella sonnei* during the acute phase (Table 48). Treatment was for 10 days duration, after which faecal samples were taken. The efficacy of the neomycin treatment was not determined as marmosets continued to die after treatment (Table 49). The isolates of organisms from these samples showed an increased resistance to neomycin. This development was known to be a hazard of treatment, but due to the severity of the outbreak, the risk had to be accepted. In recent years *Shigella sonnei* isolates from human patients have shown an increasing resistance to three or more antibiotics (Davies *et al.*, 1970). After the acute phase it has been found that the colony contains a number of symptomless excretors. Their presence has given rise to concern but as clinical signs are absent further treatment has been withheld. The appearance of these excretors is probably a result of the antibiotic treatment. Brown *et al.* (1970) showed that patients suffering from salmonellosis were more prone to become symptomless excretors after neomycin therapy than those given an inert substance. It may therefore be speculated that even in a severe outbreak treatment should be withheld.

The cause of the outbreak has not been determined. Prior to the appearance of enteritis 281 samples of faeces had been examined from the colony without the isolation of either *Shigella* or *Salmonella*. The isolation of *Shigella* species during the outbreak suggested that it may have been introduced to the colony by a human carrier or a recently introduced animal.

As no routine examinations are carried out on the faeces of staff, all five technicians responsible for the husbandry of the monkey colonies were screened but no pathogens were isolated. The primate food was prepared by other technicians but it was felt that if the organism had been introduced by the food the disease would have been seen in monkeys other than marmosets and tamarins. Five weeks before the outbreak 25 animals were introduced into the colony. During this time only one faecal sample was obtained from each cage and it is therefore highly probable that a mildly infected animal in this batch remained undetected for the reasons discussed. The source of the *Shigella sonnei* was not traced, and it was thought probable that the animals became colonized through human contacts on their arrival in the United Kingdom. Carpenter (1968) studied the isolates of *Shigella* species obtained from the intestines of freshly imported monkeys and found that 90% were *Shigella flexneri* and 3·8% were *Shigella sonnei*. This contrasted with the human situation in the United Kingdom where 98% of isolates are *Shigella sonnei* and only 2% are *Shigella flexneri*. On this evidence it was concluded that *Shigella flexneri* infections were contracted outside the UK whilst *Shigella sonnei* infections originated once the monkeys were in this country.

At the present time no monkeys are dying, but a few are excreting *Shigella sonnei* in their faeces. Microbiological testing of faeces is being continued and all isolates of the pathogen are being subjected to antibiotic sensitivity testing.

The disease outbreak in squirrel monkeys followed a somewhat different course from any in the other species of monkey in that no clinical signs were present other than diarrhoea. Various antibiotics were administered in an attempt to treat the animals as they were on a long term 2 year experiment. The experiment involved a slow growing neurotropic virus, the predictability of which was not known and which may well have been involved in the aetiology of the disease. However, when control uninoculated animals began to die before virus inoculated monkeys it was felt that the virus was not involved with the disease.

In the absence of a laboratory diagnosis and the loss of 14 animals it was arranged that the remaining monkeys would be taken to the Microbiological Research Establishment at Porton. Once on their premises the monkeys thrived and all tests gave normal results. A careful comparison was made of the methods of husbandry used at this centre and at Porton and it was concluded that some aspect of environmental control was responsible. It was known that a few days before the first cases of illness were observed, the temperature of the rooms housing the monkeys had suddenly dropped 10°C on two separate occasions. This may have triggered the outbreak, as it is well known that squirrel monkeys are severely stressed by rapid temperature drops.

A great deal of time was spent during the $2\frac{1}{2}$ years reported in this chapter, examining faeces collected from the three primate colonies. The majority of specimens did not yield any pathogenic bacteria but this finding was reassuring as it was essential to know that the colonies were free from infection. When outbreaks of disease occurred the additional samples taken aided diagnosis, particularly the choice of antibiotics following laboratory antibiotic sensitivity tests.

It may be concluded that regular screening of sub-human primate faeces should be carried out and that clinical examinations should be made, especially whilst newly arrived primates are in isolation.

9

Dogs and Farm Animals

The Diagnosis of Post-operative Infections in Dogs

Introduction

A large number of dogs have been held at the Centre for use in experiments involving major surgery. One group has been used for experimental orthopaedic surgery involving the transplantation of the knee joint (Porter and Hill, 1973) and another group for cardiovascular surgery (Cross *et al.*, 1975), involving chronic cannulation of blood vessels, and implantation of electronic monitoring devices within the thorax with leads brought to the surface.

Materials and Methods

Animals

Of the 106 dogs used for orthopaedic surgery, 81 were beagles and 25 were greyhounds.

Cardiovascular surgery involved 26 dogs of several different breeds; 11 were beagles, 4 labradors, 2 alsatians, 2 boxers and 7 crossbred dogs.

The surgery was performed in the Animal House operating theatre suite under strict aseptic conditions.

Methods

Orthopaedic Surgery

Specimens were collected either from the living animal or at subsequent autopsy.

Swabs were obtained from surgical incision lines when these became infected. They were cultured on blood agar plates both aerobically and anaerobically and inoculated into Robertson's cooked meat medium. All media were incubated at 37°C for 18 h. If there was no growth all media were reincubated for a further 24 h. Sub-cultures of the cooked meat were made on two blood agar plates if growth was observed and incubation was carried out as above. Any organisms recovered were identified according to Cowan and Steel (1966). In addition antibiotic sensitivity tests were performed on diagnostic sensitivity test agar with the addition of 7·5% lysed blood.

After surgery the dogs were retained for periods of up to 2 years after which they were sacrificed. A *post mortem* examination of the operative site was made in each case and a swab taken of the joint observing full aseptic precautions. This was then treated as described above except that no sensitivity tests were performed.

In some cases the pins holding the joint were removed for microbiological culture. These were placed in dextrose peptone water and incubated at 37°C for 18 h. If growth was present sub-cultures were made on to a blood agar plate which was incubated at 37°C for up to 48 h.

Cardiovascular Surgery

Specimens were taken from a variety of sites including blood, faeces, wounds and exudates (Cross *et al.*, 1975). Blood was incubated in special blood culture bottles containing 7 ml nutrient broth and 0·05% "liquoid" (sodium polyanethol sulphonate). Sub-cultures were made on to blood agar at weekly intervals for 2 weeks. Specimens from wounds and exudates were plated on to two blood agar plates, one incubated aerobically, the other anaerobically. A portion of each specimen was also inoculated into Robertson's cooked meat medium. After 48 h incubation or earlier if growth was observed, sub-cultures were made on to two blood agar plates.

Studies were performed in an effort to trace the source of the infection. A bacteriological survey of the faeces of all dogs in the kennels was carried out. Fresh samples were collected and inoculated on to deoxycholate citrate agar and into selenite F. Swabs were taken of many areas in the kennels including the drains, walls, taps, hose pipe and disinfectant baths. Each swab was plated on to blood agar and incubated at 37°C for 18 h.

All dogs had indwelling catheters inserted into blood vessels during surgery and, in a small survey, five of these were removed at autopsy and examined bacteriologically. Specimens were obtained by passing a small swab into the lumen of the catheter. The swab was rubbed on to two blood agar plates, one incubated aerobically, the other anaerobically and finally the swab was placed in Robertson's cooked meat.

Results

Orthopaedic Surgery

The results are summarized in Table 54. Sixty-three swabs were taken from 60 beagle dogs when these were killed and autopsied, and 41 yielded no bacterial growth. *Staphylococcus aureus* was isolated on 11 occasions, three isolates of which were typable and belonged to phage types 29, 52, 80; 25, 29, 79, 80 and 29, 52, 79, 80, 83A respectively, but the remainder proved untypable. *Staphylococcus epidermidis* was also isolated, but the remainder of the organisms were of enteric origin. Two orthopaedic fixation pins were examined and *Staphylococcus aureus* was isolated from one of these. Wound swabs yielded *Staphylococcus aureus* and enteric organisms.

Only 27 swabs were taken from 19 greyhounds. 13 of these proved sterile. Just as in the specimens obtained from the beagles, enteric organisms and *Staphylococcus aureus* were isolated from the remainder. One isolate of staphylococcus was found to be phage type 3C, 47, 54, 55, 57. Three orthopaedic fixation pins were examined, but only one yielded *Staphylococcus aureus*. Wound swabs yielded enteric organisms and *Staphylococcus* species.

Cardiovascular Surgery

The results are displayed in Table 55 and preliminary results have been published (Cross *et al.*, 1975). Forty samples of blood were examined from 22 dogs. *Pseudomonas* species was isolated on 20 occasions. This organism was also isolated from faeces, wounds and the lumen of catheters.

Antibiotic sensitivity tests showed that isolates of *Pseudomonas* species

Table 54

Bacterial isolates obtained from dogs following orthopaedic surgery

Breed of dog	Site	Number examined	Number of isolates						
			Escherichia coli	*Staphylococcus aureus*	*Pseudomonas aeruginosa*	*Proteus* sp.	*Enterobacter* sp.	*Citrobacter* sp.	*Providence* groups
Beagle	Knee joint	63	3	11	2	2	4	—	—
	Wound	11	2	4	—	—	—	—	—
	Pin	2	—	1	—	—	—	—	—
Greyhound	Knee joint	27	3	6	—	6	1	3	2
	Wound	9	2	2	2	2	—	1	2
	Pin	3	—	1	—	—	—	—	—

Table 55

Bacterial isolates obtained from dogs following cardiovascular surgery

Site	Number examined	Number of isolates				
		Clostridium welchii	*Pseudomonas* sp.	*Pseudomonas aeruginosa*	*Escherichia coli*	*Enterobacter* sp.
Blood	40	1	11	12	2	2
Faeces	4	—	2	—	1	—
Liver	1	1	1	—	—	—
Wound	6	1	1	—	2	—
Lung	2	—	—	—	2	—

Table 56

Sensitivity of isolates of Pseudomonas from cases of gram negative septicaemia

		Antimicrobial agent															
		Tetracycline	Chloramphenicol	Cephaloridine	Erythromycin	Penicillin	Ampicillin	Streptomycin	Tylosin	Chlortetracycline	Colistin methane sulphonate	Furazolidone	Neomycin	Oxytetracycline	Septrin[a]	Carbenicillin	Gentamicin
Cassidy	*Pseudomonas* sp.	R	R	R	R	R	R	R	R	R	S	R	R	R	R	R	—
Watson	*P. aeruginosa*	R	R	R	R	R	R	R	R	R	R	R	R	R	R	S	—
Sundance	*P. aeruginosa*	R	R	R	R	R	R	R	R	R	S	R	S	R	R	R	—
Thorpe	*Pseudomonas* sp.	R	R	R	R	R	R	R	R	R	S	R	R	R	R	S	—
Heath	*Pseudomonas* sp.	R	R	R	R	R	R	R	R	R	S	R	R	R	R	R	—
Midge	*P. aeruginosa*	R	R	R	R	R	R	R	R	R	R	R	R	R	R	S	S
Annexus	*P. aeruginosa*	R	R	R	R	R	R	R	R	R	S	R	R	R	R	R	S
Amon	*Pseudomonas* sp.	R	R	R	R	R	R	R	R	R	S	R	S	R	R	R	S
Sonnet	*P. aeruginosa*	R	R	R	R	R	R	R	R	R	S	R	S	R	R	R	S

[a] Sulfamethoxazole/Trimethoprim.
R, Resistant; S, Sensitive.
—, not tested.

isolated from post-operative animals, were very resistant to these agents (Table 56). The organism was always sensitive to gentamicin and nearly all were sensitive to colistin methane sulphonate. A few isolates were sensitive to neomycin and carbenicillin.

From the faecal survey of normal dogs it was found that nine out of 16 dogs carried *Pseudomonas aeruginosa* in their faeces (Table 57). When these isolates were tested against antibiotics *in vitro* the sensitivity patterns (Table 58) were similar to that described above.

Table 57

Number of isolates of *Pseudomonas aeruginosa* obtained from normal dog faeces

Breed	Number of isolates/ number of dogs examined
Greyhound	4/5
Beagle	2/7
Crossbred	2/2
Labrador	1/2

Discussion

The number of samples collected from a total of 136 dogs was larger than anticipated. This situation arose mainly because the animals were involved in major surgical procedures and unfortunately were subject to infection, mainly localized in dogs used for orthopaedic surgery, but systemic in the cardiovascular group.

Sixty-six per cent of the routine specimens from beagles and 50% from greyhounds used for orthopaedic surgery proved to be sterile. This was to be expected, as the majority of these specimens were taken from dogs 2 years after surgery where there was no overt sign of infection. From the other cases, *Staphylococcus aureus* was frequently isolated. Great care was taken when each specimen was obtained so it was felt that the organisms present were not the result of contamination. Charnley (1972) reported the isolation of *Staphylococcus aureus* and enteric organisms from human hip joint replacement patients and it would appear that this animal model is subject to the same risk of infection as the human patient. It was also apparent that the greyhounds were infected by more species of organisms than the beagles. No reason for this was known except that

Table 58

Sensitivity to antimicrobial agents of *Pseudomonas aeruginosa* isolated from faeces of normal dogs

Breed of dog	Number of isolates	Number of isolates sensitive																
		Chloramphenicol	Cephaloridine	Erythromycin	Kanamycin	Penicillin	Ampicillin	Streptomycin	Tetracycline	Tylosin	Chlortetracycline	Colistin methane sulphonate	Furazolidone	Neomycin	Oxytetracycline	Gentamicin	Septrin[a]	Carbenicillin
Greyhound	5	0	0	0	0	0	0	0	0	0	0	3	0	4	0	5	0	3
Beagle	2	0	0	0	0	0	0	0	0	0	0	1	0	0	0	2	0	1
Crossbred	2	0	0	0	0	0	0	0	0	0	0	2	0	1	0	2	0	1

[a] Sulfamethoxazole Trimethoprim.

later, as part of the studies on dogs subjected to cardiovascular surgery, the faeces of greyhounds were found to be colonized by more species of organisms than beagles.

Staphylococcus aureus was frequently isolated from beagle wound infections whereas enteric organisms were more frequently isolated from wound infections in greyhounds.

A great deal of work was performed with the specimens obtained from dogs involved in cardiovascular surgery. The complicating factor following surgery was a Gram negative septicaemia as reported by Cross *et al.* (1975). The causative organism was found to be *Pseudomonas* species and it was isolated from blood samples as well as intravascular catheters (Table 59).

Table 59

Isolates of bacteria obtained from catheters and guidewires following cardiovascular surgery

Dog name	Site	Isolate
Cassidy	Guide wire	*Pseudomonas* sp.
Amigo	Catheter lumen	*Pseudomonas* sp.
Thorpe	Catheter lumen	*Pseudomonas* sp.
Wilson	Arterial catheter	No isolates
	Jugular catheter	*Escherichia coli*

The survey of canine faeces showed that this organism was carried by many of the dogs. When isolated from normal dogs, *Pseudomonas* was found to be resistant to antibiotics which suggested that a subsequent infection would be difficult to treat.

When the isolates of *Pseudomonas aeruginosa* obtained from sick dogs were typed, only two types were differentiated but these did not match the types obtained from sources within the kennels. The source of the infections has not been traced but treatment with an antibiotic regime rationally based on the laboratory findings, has meant that the experiments are now not frustrated by septicaemia.

The Microbiological Examination of Farm Animals for Enteric Pathogens

Introduction

Small numbers of farm animals have been held for long term antiserum production and experimental surgery. These animals presented a hazard to the facility because of the danger of the introduction of enteric organisms, particularly *Salmonella* species. For this reason it was decided that this group of animals should be regularly checked for the presence of pathogenic enteric organisms.

Materials and Methods

Faecal samples were obtained from goats, pigs, sheep and calves as shown in Table 60. Faeces were obtained for the first 3 days following arrival of the animal at the Centre and further samples were collected at monthly intervals.

The samples were plated on to deoxycholate citrate agar and into selenite F.

Table 60

Number of samples of faeces examined from farm animals

Species	Number of samples
Goats	48
Pigs	62
Sheep	15
Calves	8

Results

One hundred and thirty-three samples of faeces were examined but at no time were either *Salmonella* or *Shigella* species isolated.

Discussion

When the laboratory work was divided into various categories before the screening programme was commenced, it was anticipated that large animals would not provide many specimens, although it is now realized that the importance of this area of the programme was underestimated.

In numbers, large animals held within the facility, are the smallest groups of experimental animals. However, the experiments in which they become involved are expensive and far more time consuming, both in research workers' time and husbandry, than those experiments using mice. Additionally, each animal forms an experiment, whereas several mice may be used for one experiment. Hence if illness causes the death of a large animal the scientific work is severely frustrated.

The presence within the Animal House of farm animals was considered to be a possible source of the introduction of enteric pathogens into the building, because of the known carriage by these animals of *Salmonella* species. In the event it has been found that no farm animals have ever carried *Salmonella* species and this is probably a reflection of the quality of the suppliers of these animals. On balance the work involved in screening faecal samples has been justified. With the techniques used the procedures are neither time consuming nor costly and unlike other workers (Caraway *et al.*, 1968) surveillance will be continued.

It may be concluded that the screening of large animals to determine their microbiological status, in relation to enteric organisms, is essential in a facility with many species of animals. Further, when clinical cases of illness are detected every effort should be made to determine the causal agent and suitable treatment.

10

Discussion

The various studies reported in this book spanned a $2\frac{1}{2}$ year period of operation of an animal health and quality control programme. At the outset it was considered essential that such a programme should start and the results obtained have justified this opinion. Unfortunately the literature does not contain details of similar schemes and hence comparison is impossible. However, there are references to surveys of animal health and these will be considered in relation to the system at this Centre.

Literature searches revealed reports of two large surveys of animal health in laboratory animal colonies (Lane-Petter *et al.,* 1955; Seamer *et al.,* 1967). Both were carried out by the analysis of questionnaires and hence did not deal in any detail with techniques or interpretation of data. They clearly revealed a lack of awareness of the problems of disease in laboratory animals; for example in the latter survey one laboratory reported that they lost no animals due to clinical disease which is patently absurd and could only be a failure to recognize disease. In 1960, Izard and Roberts published details of the laboratory quality control programme that was set up when the Laboratory Animals Centre was moved to Carshalton. In those early days, the extent of the investigations was rather limited, although they did include in their programme, disinfectant testing and other aspects of animal house hygiene. As has already been detailed, the Clinical Research Centre scheme examined several aspects of animal house hygiene and environmental control and obviously any programme concerned with quality control must include them. Melby (1970) was the only publication traced of American origin, and he called for a "seal of approval" quality of laboratory animals. However, although it is known that laboratory animal quality control is now practised in the USA details of the programmes do not appear to have been published.

Since these publications were located and work commenced, there has been a vast increase in the awareness of the problems of laboratory animal disease and the effect of the disease on experimental results. Southee (1974) described the role of diagnostic bacteriology in an animal house and gave brief details of the examinations undertaken. The awareness of the problems prompted an editorial in the *Lancet* (1974) in which it was stated that "so-called specified or specific pathogen-free (SPF) animals—yield results which are intrinsically more reliable than those from experiments on disease-ridden stock" and later on in the article "and the control of disease still falls short of what is both desirable and possible". These two quotes sum up the thinking behind the programme at this Centre. Parallel with this, an editorial was published in an American publication, *Lab Animal* (1974), which again made out a case for the inclusion of quality control and diagnostic services in every animal facility. The editorial suggested three areas in which laboratory work should be performed; in the diagnosis of disease and quality control, in specialized teaching and finally in research into diseases. White (1974) published details of his work on quality control and stated that "if an investigator using animals thinks he doesn't need the support of a diagnostic laboratory, he is just kidding himself".

It must be stressed that these latter publications have appeared 2 years or more after the start of the programme at this centre and it is interesting to note that they confirm the decisions made in early 1972.

Before considering the broader aspects of the programme some comparisons may be made with the above publications. The papers by Lane-Petter *et al.* (1955) and Seamer *et al.* (1967) both concluded that insufficient attention was given to recording the details of disease outbreaks. With this in mind, a system employing punched cards was devised which has enabled full details of all sections of the programme to be permanently recorded, combined with easy retrieval of data.

The only survey to deal specifically with diseases and their causal agents was that of Seamer and Chesterman (1967). They received 40 replies to their questionnaire and when analysed, the findings may be compared with the results obtained from this survey at the Clinical Research Centre.

Pasteurella pneumotropica was reported to have been associated with abscessation of many sites, whereas at this Centre the only clinical condition associated with this organism has been mouse eye infections (Needham and Cooper, 1975). Mouse mites were found on many conventionally housed mice and they proved difficult to control. But, from Seamer and Chesterman's survey, this might be expected as in 1967 20% of establishments were infested by mites and hence any unit purchasing mice must be exposed to the hazard of mite infestation being introduced on animals brought into the facility. This risk can be reduced by ensuring that mice bought for use in research work are category *** or higher in the Laboratory Animals Centre Accreditation Scheme as these animals must be free from ectoparasites. Seamer and Chesterman expressed surprise when few establishments reported colonization of mice by the nematode *Syphacia obvelata*, but this too, has been the case in mice at this Centre. What is more, only one batch of mice from a commercial source was found to be colonized by this endoparasite although many were examined from eight different suppliers. This would suggest that *Syphacia obvelata* is not widely distributed amongst mouse colonies.

The programme was designed to protect the Animal House from the risk of contamination by pathogens and to ensure that the animals bred were of a consistently high standard. The greatest danger was presented by the large numbers of animals bought from commercial sources when the facility was first opened. It was thought essential that incoming animals were screened even though the breeders were accredited by the Laboratory Animals Centre. The accreditation scheme only provides for the twice yearly examination of breeding colonies which is unlikely to give early warning of microbiological contamination of a colony although it has undoubtedly imposed far higher standards on commercial suppliers and upgraded their stock. For this reason the screening of incoming stock formed a prominent part of the programme and has revealed three breeders' colonies whose animals if brought into the Animal House, would have caused contamination. One was infested with mites, mice from another carried a heavy *Syphacia obvelata* burden and the other breeder sold mice infected with *Mycoplasma* species. Clearly, mice from these sources were unsuitable and hence further purchases were not made. It may be asked why infections such as the above, occur in breeders' colonies, especially when the breeders are encouraged to maintain quality control of their premises. Unfortunately, some breeders maintain only very low levels of control which are quite insufficient to ensure the early detection of infections. In our experience the disappointing quality of many purchased animals emphasized the necessity for the purchaser to screen any animals on arrival, before they are mixed with animals already in stock.

When the Animal House was opened it was decided that a barrier maintained breeding colony would be built up to supply up to 90% of the rodents required within the Clinical Research Centre. It has been shown that as the supply of animals from this unit increased, a steady improvement in health status of the whole Animal House colony took place. When the programme was commenced, research workers frequently requested assistance due to disease problems in their animals. As time passed, the number of requests diminished until, as at present, very little help is needed and rodents are known to be of a high standard. It was also noted that the numbers of organisms isolated from sentinel mice decreased as the numbers of mice of barrier unit origin in each room increased, confirming the improved health status within the building. With this improvement it was seen that respiratory infections decreased and diarrhoea was no longer observed in litters of mice.

The quality control of the barrier unit did not yield any surprising results. The large numbers of animals tested have shown a remarkably stable microbiological status. Only one organism, *Staphylococcus aureus*, entered the unit as a contaminant and was responsible for overt disease. This could constitute, by definition, a breakdown of the barrier unit, but was not regarded as such because no interference with the breeding and subsequent use of the animals in experiments occurred as it was noted after issue from the unit the organism was quickly replaced by the organisms present in each conventional room.

The provision of a diagnostic service, both for the research worker and as an aid to animal management decisions has entailed a great deal of work. This was due in the main to outbreaks of enteric disease in the primate colonies, particularly the outbreak of shigellosis in the marmosets. It was impossible to accurately forecast where disease outbreaks were likely to occur, but the work carried out has shown that White (1974) was correct in stating that a diagnostic laboratory is essential to the research worker. It is difficult to judge the total benefit of this service as in many cases the diagnostic tests were performed following a *post mortem* examination. However, the value of the service was clearly illustrated in dogs. These are extremely expensive to purchase as well as maintain so that post-operative infections, sometimes fatal, were particularly costly and research projects were disrupted. The speedy laboratory diagnosis of the causative organism followed by appropriate treatment meant that in many cases the experiment could proceed without delay.

The detailed organization of the animal health and quality control programme has been described. When the scheme was devised the likely numbers of specimens to be examined could only be predicted. However, experience has shown that the scheme has been able to cope with the numbers and variety of specimens, although areas of work have had to be modified. The biggest of these involved the frequency of sampling of the various colonies of animals and the size of sample examined. When work was commenced it was possible for one technologist, with occasional help, to screen the colonies of animals at short regular intervals. However, as more research workers were appointed to the Clinical Research Centre, the laboratory received more specimens, until, with no additional staff available it became clear that a realistic sampling frequency had to be arranged. This involved a reduction in the frequency of sampling of each individual colony although not a reduction in the sample size. It was felt that this was justified because the results obtained could be compared with the data already accumulated.

It must be admitted that screening a large colony of animals could become an open handed commitment, probably with the law of diminishing returns operating, so a limited programme must be continued including screening of marker animals, rather than total microbiological analysis of each specimen.

The animal health scheme, as set out in this book, can easily be carried out by one experienced technologist with minimal assistance and it is now proposed to expand certain areas of the scheme in the light of the results obtained. Chief of these will be the microbiological screening of incoming stock. It is known that some institutes are infected by Ectromelia virus and others by mouse mange. A policy has therefore been instituted whereby all incoming stock is held in an isolation area, and where possible, 10% are removed and microbiologically screened. When the results are known, the veterinary pathologist decides whether the animals are permitted to enter the main colonies. This policy has already detected cases of infection, which, if the animals had been permitted to join the colony on their arrival, would have posed a severe health threat.

It has been concluded that it is essential to maintain a health control scheme in the Animal House and that this scheme should involve the regular microbiological monitoring of the breeding unit, the environment including equipment and all incoming animals. Early detection of cases of clinical illness is important and close cooperation between the veterinary and laboratory staff will ensure that diagnosis can be achieved and the appropriate treatment administered promptly.

References

Arya, S. C., Verghese, A., Agarwal, D. S. and Pal, S. C. (1973). Shigellosis in rhesus monkeys in quarantine. *Lab. Anim.,* **7,** 101.

Aserkoff, B. and Bennett, J. V. (1969). Effect of antibiotic therapy in acute salmonellosis on the faecal excretion of salmonellae. *New Engl. J. Med.,* **281,** 636.

Bach, F. W., Fülscher, J. and Harnack (1931). Uber eine durch Affen verursachte Ruhrepidemie. *Veröff Med-Verw.,* **34,** 61.

Baermann, G. and Halberstaedter, L. (1906). Experimentelle Hauttuberkulose bei Affen. *Berl. klin. Wschr.,* **43,** 199.

Baker, F. J. (1969). "Handbook of Bacteriological Technique". Second edn, Butterworth & Co., London.

Bell, D. P. and Elmes, P. C. (1969). Effects of certain organisms associated with chronic respiratory disease on S.P.F. and conventional rats. *J. med. Microbiol.,* **2,** 511.

Blackmore, D. K. and Francis, R. A. (1970). The apparent transmission of Staphylococci of human origin to laboratory animals. *J. comp. Path.* **80,** 645.

Blackmore, D. K. and Hill, A. C. (1972a). The Isolation and Identification of Bacteria and Mycoplasma pathogenic to Laboratory Animals. *In* "Safety in Microbiology" (D. A. Shapton and R. G. Board, eds). Academic Press, London and New York.

Blackmore, D. K., Guillon, J. C. and Schwanzer, V. (1972b). "The Viruses of Laboratory Rodents and Lagomorphs". (D. K. Blackmore, ed.) ICLA Virus Reference Laboratory Sub-Committee. Published by BVA Editorial Services.

Bleby, J. (1976). "Specific Pathogen Free Animals". The UFAW Handbook on the Care and Management of Laboratory Animals. Fifth edn. Churchill Livingstone, Edinburgh and London.

Boddie, G. F. (1962). "Diagnostic Methods in Veterinary Medicine". Fifth edn, Oliver and Boyd, Edinburgh and London.

Bouley, G. and Stupfel, M. (1970). Facteurs sexuels et resistance aux toxiques, virus et bacteries chez les Mammiferes. *Bull. Inst. Nat. Sante Rech. Med.*, **25,** 1249.

Bouley, G., Dubreuil, A., Pruliere, D. and Bouley, M. (1974). Sex factors in airborne infection: comparative susceptibility of male and female non-immunized mice to aerosolized *Pasteurella multocida. Lab. Anim.*, **8,** 9.

Brandish, J. M. and Willis, A. T. (1970). Observations on the coagulase and deoxyribonuclease tests for staphylococci. *J. Med. Lab. Technol.*, **27,** 355.

Brennan, P. C., Fritz, T. E. and Flynn, R. J. (1965). *Pasteurella pneumotropica:* cultural and biochemical characteristics and its association with disease in laboratory animals. *Lab. Anim. Care,* **15,** 307.

Brennan, P. C., Fritz, T. E. and Flynn, R. J. (1969a). Role of *Pasteurella pneumotropica* and *Mycoplasma pulmonis* in murine pneumonia. *J. Bact.*, **97,** 337.

Brennan, P. C., Fritz, T. E. and Flynn, R. J. (1969b). Murine pneumonia: a review of the etiologic agents. *Lab. Animal Care,* **19,** 360.

Brown, E. H., Laing Brown, G., Latham Brown, D., Edmond, R. T. D., Galpine, J. F., Jamieson, S. R., Lamb, S. G., Lambert, J. P., McKendrick, G. D. W., Medlock, J. M. and Vahrman, J. (1970). The effect of neomycin in non-invasive Salmonella infections of the gastrointestinal tract. *Lancet,* **ii,** 1159.

Brown, L. R., Handler, S., Allen, S. S., Shea, C., Wheatcroft, M. G. and Frome, W. J. (1973). Oral microbial profile of the marmoset. *J. dent. Res.*, **52,** 815.

Bywater, J. E. C., Hartley, E. G., Rutty, D. A. and Ackerley, E. T. (1962). Observations on the intradermal palpebral tuberculin test and subsequent autopsy findings in monkeys. *Vet. Rec.*, **74,** 1414.

Caraway, B. L., Estes, R. R., Neola, P. M. and Thornton, O. W. (1968). Results of screening for *Shigella* and other enteric bacteria in Rhesus Monkeys during quarantine. *Lab. Anim. Care,* **18,** 568.

Carpenter, K. P. and Cooke, E. R. N. (1965). An attempt to find Shigellae in wild primates. *J. comp. Path.*, **75,** 201.

Carpenter, K. P. (1968). Human and simian shigellosis. In "Some diseases of Animals Communicable to man in Britain" (O. Graham-Jones, ed.). Pergamon, Oxford.

Carthew, P. and Verstraete, A. (1978). A serological survey of accredited breeding colonies in the United Kingdom for common rodent viruses. *Lab. Anim.*, **12,** 29.

Casillo, S. and Blackmore, D. K. (1972). Uterine infections caused by bacteria and mycoplasma in mice and rats. *J. comp. Path.*, **82,** 477.

Chaffee, P. S. (1972). Zoonoses considerations. *In* "American Association of Zoo Veterinarians Annual Proceedings". 1972 Houston and 1973 Colombus.

Chanock, R. M., Hayflick, L. and Barile, M. F. (1962). Growth on artificial medium of an agent associated with atypical pneumonia and its identification as a PPLO. *Proc. natn. Acad. Sci., Washington,* **48,** 41.

Charnley, J. (1972). Post-operative infection after total hip replacement with special reference to air contamination in the operating room. *Clin. Ortho. Related Res.*, **87**, 167.

Chattopadhyay, B. and Pilford, J. B. (1976). The effect of prolonged incubation of Selenite F broth on the rate of isolation of *Salmonella* from faeces. *Med. Lab. Sci.*, **33**, 191.

Clarke, M. C., Taylor, R. J., Hall, G. A. and Jones, P. W. (1978). The occurrence in mice of facial and mandibular abscesses associated with *Staphylococcus aureus*. *Lab. Anim.*, **12**, 121.

Coid, C. R. (1969). Management in relation to safety in a laboratory primate unit. *In* "Hazards of Handling Simians". *Lab. Anim. Handb.*, **4.**

Constantine, M. L. (1972). Effects of insecticides on acariasis in mice. *Lab. Anim.*, **6**, 279.

Cook, R. (1953a). The naturally occurring diseases of laboratory animals and practical measures for the control of these diseases. *J. Med. Lab. Technol.*, **11**, 30.

Cook, R. (1953b). Murine mange: the control of *Myocoptes musculinus* and *Myobia musculi* infestations. *Br. Vet. J.*, **109**, 113.

Cook, R. (1969). Simian shigellosis. *In* "Hazards of Handling Simians", *Lab. Anim. Handb.*, **4.**

Cooper, J. E. and Needham, J. R. (1976a). Investigation of alopecia following sulphur rolling of mice. *Lab. Anim.*, **10**, 349.

Cooper, J. E. and Needham, J. R. (1976b). An outbreak of shigellosis in laboratory marmosets and tamarins (Family: Callithricidae). *J. Hyg. Camb.*, **76**, 415.

Cowan, S. T. and Steel, K. J. (1966). "Manual for the Identification of Medical Bacteria". Cambridge University Press.

Cross, M. R., Cooper, J. E. and Needham, J. R. (1975). Observations on a post-operative septicaemia in experimental dogs with particular reference to *Pseudomonas aeruginosa*. *J. comp. Path.*, **85**, 445.

Davies, G. O. (1962). "Gaiger and Davies' Veterinary Pathology and Bacteriology", Fourth edn, Bailliere, Tindall and Cox, London.

Davies, J. R., Farrant, W. N. and Uttley, A. H. (1970). Antibiotic resistance of *Shigella sonnei*. *Lancet*, **ii**, 1157.

Davis, R. (1957). Control of the myocoptic mange mite *Myocoptes musculinus* (Koch) on laboratory mice. *J. econ. Ent.*, **50**, 695.

Deinhardt, F., Holmes, A. W., Devine, J. and Deinhardt, J. (1967). Marmosets as laboratory animals. *Lab. Anim. Care*, **17**, 48.

Dixon, J. M. S. (1965). Effect of antibiotic treatment on duration of excretion of *Salmonella typhimurium* by children. *Br. Mrd. J.*, **2**, 1343.

Editorial (1974). *Lab. Animal*, **3**, No. 3, 10.

Editorial (1974). Quality of laboratory animals. *Lancet*, **ii**, 389.

Fernando, N. I. and Heath, R. B. (1971a). Studies of the Heat Lability of Mouse Anti-Sendai Virus Immune Sera. *Arch. ges. Virusforsch.*, **34**, 295.

Fernando, N. I. and Heath, R. B. (1971b). A study of Non-specific Inhibition of Paramyxoviruses by Animal Sera. *Indian J. med. Res.*, **59**, 537.

Fisk, A. (1940). The technique of the Coagulase Test for Staphylococci. *Br. J. exp. Path.*, **21**, 311.
Flynn, R. J. (1955). Ectoparasites in mice. *Pro. Anim. Care Panel,* **6,** 75.
Flynn, R. J., Brennan, P. C., and Fritz, T. E. (1965). Pathogen status of commercially produced laboratory mice. *Lab. Anim. Care,* **15,** 440.
Galton, M. (1963). Myobic mange in mice leading to skin ulceration and amyloidosis. *Amer. J. Path.,* **43,** 855.
Gambles, R. M. (1952). *Myocoptes musculinus* (Koch) and *Myobia musculi* (Shrank) two species of mite commonly parasitising the laboratory mouse. *Br. Vet. J.,* **108,** 194.
Green, C. J. and Needham, J. R. (1974a). Control of mange mites in a large mouse colony. *Lab. Anim.,* **8,** 245.
Green, C. J. and Needham, J. R. (1974b). A simple technique for sulphur dressing mice. *Lab. Anim.,* **8,** 327.
Green, C. J., Needham, J. R. and Cooper, J. E. (1975). *Lactobacillus* sp. isolates from mouse livers: saprophyte or potential pathogen? *Lab. Anim.,* **9,** 149.
Guyton, A. C. (1947). Measurements of the respiratory volumes of laboratory animals. *Am. J. Physiol.,* **150,** 70.
Hale, P. and Hill, A. C. (1973). The recovery of *Lactobacillus* sp. from the livers of healthy mice. *Lab. Anim.,* **7,** 119.
Haltalin, K. C., Kusmiesz, H. T., Hinton, L. V. and Nelson, J. D. (1972). Treatment of acute diarrhoea in outpatients. *Am. J. Dis. Child.,* **124,** 554.
Heath, R. B. (1971). Personal communication.
Hentges, D. J. (1967). Inhibition of *Shigella flexneri* by the normal intestinal flora. I. Mechanisms of inhibition by *Klebsiella. J. Bact.,* **93,** 1369.
Heston, W. E. and Deringer, M. K. (1948). Hereditary renal disease and amyloidosis in mice. *Archs. Path.,* **46,** 49.
Hill, A. (1966). The bacteriological control of an S.P.F. unit. *J. Inst. Anim. Techns.,* **17,** 133.
Hill, M. J. (1969). Protection of mice against infection by *Staphylococcus aureus. J. Med. Microbiol.,* **2,** 1.
Izard, J. L. and Roberts, M. L. (1960). Laboratory control of infection in a small animal colony. *J. Anim. Assoc.,* **11,** 67.
Jacobs, S. I., Willis, A. T. and Goodburn, G. (1964). Pigment Production and Enzymic Activity of Staphylococci: The Differentiation of Pathogens from Commensals. *J. Path. Bact.,* **87,** 151.
Jafary, M. H. and Burke, G. J. (1970). Antibiotics and salmonella excretors. *Br. Med. J.* **2,** 605.
Jarvis, J. D. and Wynne, C. D. (1969). A short survey of the reliability of deoxyribonuclease as an adjunct in the determination of staphylococcal pathogenicity. *J. Med. Lab. Technol.,* **26,** 131.
Jones, J. B., Estes, P. C. and Jordan, A. E. (1972). *Proteus mirabilis* infection in a mouse colony. *J. Am. vet. med. Ass.,* **161,** 661.
Kalter, S. S. and Heberling, R. L. (1969). The Study of Simian Viruses. *WHO Chronicle,* **23,** 112.
Keeble, S. A. (1968). B Virus Infection in Man and Monkey. *In* "Some

Diseases of Animals Communicable to Man in Britain". (O. Graham-Jones, ed.). Pergamon: Oxford.

Lane-Petter, W., Barber, A. P. and King, H. J. (1955). Survey of laboratory animals in Great Britain. *Br. Vet. J.*, **111,** 282.

Lexomboon, U., Mansuwan, P., Duangmani, C., Benjadol, P. and Talmage McMinn, M. (1972). Clinical evaluation of Co-trimaxazole and Furazolidone in the treatment of shigellosis in children. *Br. Med. J.* **3,** p. 23.

Lindsey, J. R., Hardy, P. H., Baker, H. J. and Melby, E. C. (1971). Observations on shigellosis and development of multiply resistant shigellas in *Macaca mulatta. Lab. Aninl. Sci.*, **21,** 832.

Madden, A. H., Tozolski, A. H. and Sweetman, H. L. (1954). Control of *Myobia musculi* (Shrank) and *Myocoptes musculinus* (Koch) on laboratory mice. *J. econ. Ent.*, **47,** 442.

Mann, P. H. and Bjotvedt, G. (1966). Altre informazioni riguardanti la tipizzazione batteriofagica dei ceppi di stafilococchi coagulasi positivi isolati da varie specie di animali domestici, selvatici e di laboratorie. *Arch. Vet. Ital.* **17,** 357.

Melby, E. C. (1970). Letter to the Editor, *Lab. Anim. Care*, **20,** 583.

Miles, A. A. (1951). The mouse pathogenicity and toxicity of *Proteus vulgaris. J. gen. Microbiol.*, **5,** 307.

Morrison, S. M., Fair, J. F. and Kennedy, K. K. (1961). *Staphylococcus aureus* in Domestic Animals. *Pub. Hth. Rep.*, **76,** 673.

Needham, J. R. (1974). A study of the coagulase and deoxyribonuclease tests applied to staphylococci from non-human sources. *J. Med. Lab. Technol.*, **31,** 141.

Needham, J. R. (1975). The laboratory investigation of an outbreak of diarrhoea in Rhesus Monkeys. *J. Inst. Animal Technic.*, **26,** 17.

Needham, J. R. and Cooper, J. E. (1975). An eye infection in laboratory mice associated with *Pasteurella pneumotropica. Lab. Animals*, **9,** 197.

Needham, J. R. (1977). The collection of animal faeces for laboratory examination. *J. Inst. Anim. Tech.*, **28,** 63.

Needham, J. R. and Cooper, J. E. (1976). Bulbourethral gland infections in mice associated with *Staphylococcus aureus. Lab. Anim.*, **10,** 311.

Needham, J. R. (1978). The control of mange mites (*Myocoptes musculinus* and *Myobia musculi*) in a conventional mouse colony. *J. Inst. Anim. Techns.*, **29,** 1.

Oldham, J. N. (1967). *In* "Pathology of Laboratory Rats and Mice" (E. Cotchin and F. J. C. Roe, eds) Chap. 20. Blackwell, Oxford and Edinburgh.

Owen, D. (1972). *In* "Common Parasites of Laboratory Rodents and Lagomorphs". Her Majesty's Stationery Office, London.

Page, K. W. (1974). Automatic control of guinea-pig lice with a synergised pyrethrins aerosol. *Vet. Rec.*, **94,** 254.

Parker, J. C., Tennant, R. W., Ward, T. G. and Rowe, W. P. (1965). Virus studies with Germfree Mice. I. Preparation of Serologic Diagnostic Reagents and Survey of Germfree and Monocontaminated Mice for Indigenous Murine Viruses. *J. natn. Cancer Inst.*, **34,** 371.

Parker, M. T. (1974). Personal communication.

Peace, T. and Soave, O. (1971). Antibodies in germfree mice against mouse viruses following exposure to infected mice. *Lab. Animal Sci.,* **21,** 537.

Pinkerton, M. E. (1968). Shigellosis in the baboon (*Papio* sp.). *Lab. Anim. Care,* **18,** 11.

Poiley, S. M. (1970). A survey of indigenous murine viruses in a variety of production and research animal facilities. *Lab. Anim. Care,* **20,** 643.

Porter, B. B. and Hill, R. D. (1973). Transplantation of the canine knee joint using an oesteochondral shell graft. International Congress Series No. 324.

Rewell, R. E. and Bridges, R. F. (1948). An outbreak of *Shigella flexneri* infection among Rhesus monkeys. *Mont. Bull. Minist. H.,* **1,** 25.

Ruch, T. C. (1959). "Diseases of Laboratory Primates", Chapter 3. W. B. Saunders Co., Philadelphia and London.

Sanyal, R. B. (1892). "A Handbook of the Management of Animals in Captivity in Lower Bengal". Bengal Secretariat Press, Bengal XIIV.

Schiff, L. J., Barbera, P. W., Port, C. D., Yamashiroya, H. M., Shefner, A. M. and Poiley, S. M. (1972). Enteropathogenic *Escherichia coli* infections: increasing awareness of a problem in laboratory animals. *Lab. Anim. Sci.,* **22,** 705.

Schroder, C. R. (1938). A diagnostic test for the recognition of tuberculosis in primates: a preliminary report. *Zoologica, N.Y.,* **23,** 397.

Seamer, J. and Chesterman, F. C. (1967). A survey of disease in laboratory animals. *Lab. Anim.,* **1,** 117.

Sebesteny, A. (1973). Abscesses of the bulbourethral glands of mice due to *Pasteurella pneumotropica. Lab. Anim.,* **7,** 315.

Sebesteny, A. (1974). The transmission of intestinal flagellates between mice and rats. *Lab. Anim.,* **8,** 79.

South, M. A. (1971). Enteropathogenic *Escherichia coli* disease. New developments and perspectives. *J. Paediat.,* **79,** 1.

Southee, T. (1974). The role of diagnostic bacteriology in the animal house. *J. Inst. Anim. Tech.,* **25,** 37.

Stickler, D. J. (1970). Some observations on the detection of Staphylococcal deoxyribonuclease. *J. Med. Lab. Technol.,* **27,** 83.

Stokes, E. J. (1973). Personal communication.

Stones, P. B. (1969). Incidence of tuberculosis in *Macaca mulatta* and *Cercopithecus aethiops* monkeys with special reference to the tuberculin test. *Lab. Anim. Handb.,* **4,** 11.

Takasaka, M., Honjo, S., Fujiwara, T., Hagiwara, T., Ogawa, H. and Imaizumi, K. (1964). Shigellosis in Cynomolgus monkeys (*Macaca irus*). I. Epidemiological surveys on shigella infection rate. *Jap. J. med. Sci. Biol.,* **17,** 259.

Taylor, R. J. (1974). The sterilization of a new building designed for the breeding of specific-pathogen-free animals. *J. Hyg., Camb.,* **72,** 41.

Taylor-Robinson, D., Denny, F. W., Thompson, G. W., Allison, A. C. and Mardh, P. A. (1972). Isolation of Mycoplasmas from lungs by a Perfusion Technique. *Med. Microbiol. Immunol.,* **158,** 9.

Tennant, R. W., Parker, J. C. and Ward, T. G. (1966). Respiratory virus infections of mice. *Natn. Cancer Inst. Monog.* No. 20, 93.

Thompson, G. (1975). Personal communication.

Townsend, G. H. (1969). The Grading of Commercially-Bred Laboratory Animals. *Vet. Rec.,* **85,** 225.

Tuffery, A. A. (1956). Epidemiology and laboratory mice. *Coll. Pap. Lab. Anim. Bur.,* **4,** 7.

Tuffery, A. A. (1959). The health of laboratory mice: a comparison of general health in two breeding units where different systems are employed. *J. Hyg., Camb.,* **57,** 386.

Tuffery, A. A. (1962). Health control in a mouse population. *Z. Versuchstierkunde,* **1,** 110.

Tyrrell, D. A. J. and Coid, C. R. (1970). Sendai virus infection of rats as a convenient model of acute respiratory infection. *Vet. Rec.,* **86,** 164.

Tyzzer, E. E. (1917). A fatal disease of the Japanese Waltzing mouse caused by a spore-bearing bacillus (*Bacillus piliformis,* N. s.p.). *J. med. Res.,* **37,** 307.

van Bekkum, D. W. (1970). Immunosuppressive Regimens: Hazards to Experimental Animals and Personnel. An Introduction. *In* "Infections and Immunosuppression in Subhuman Primates". (H. Balner and W. I. B. Beveridge, eds). Scandinavian University Books.

van der Veen, J., Poort, Y. and Birchfield, D. J. (1974). Study of the possible persistence of Sendai virus in mice. *Lab. Anim. Sci.,* **24,** 48.

Verstraete, A. P. (1973). Comparison of techniques for taking liver and lung samples from small rodents for bacteriological culture. *Lab. Anim.,* **7,** 189.

Walburg, H. E., Mynatt, E. I., Cosgrove, G. E., Tyndall, R. L. and Robie, D. M. (1965). Microbiological evaluation of an isolation facility for the production of Specific-Pathogen-Free Mice. *Lab. Anim. Care,* **15,** 208.

Weil, J. D., Ward, M. K. and Spertzel, R. O. (1971). Incidence of *Shigella* in conditioned rhesus monkeys (*Macaca mulatta*). *Lab. Anim. Sci.,* **21,** 434.

White, C. Y. and Fox, H. (1909). Results of tuberculin tests in monkeys at Philadelphia Zoological Garden. *Archs. inter. med.,* **4,** 517.

White, W. J. (1974). If an investigator using animals thinks he doesn't need the support of a diagnostic laboratory he is just kidding himself. *Lab. Animal,* **3,** No. 2, 31.

Appendix 1

Number of animals held at the Clinical Research Centre

Mice	*Mus musculus*	27 000
Rats	*Rattus norvegicus*	2000
Guinea-pigs	*Cavia porcellus*	300
Rabbits	*Oryctolagus cuniculus*	200
Dogs	*Canis familiaris*	30
Monkeys	*Macaca mulatta*	120
	Macaca fascicularis	
	Saguinus sp.	
	Callithrix jacchus	
Chickens	*Gallus domesticus*	12
Goats	*Capra hircus*	4
Sheep	*Ovis aries*	4
Pigs	*Sus scrofa domestica*	12

Appendix 2

Level 3

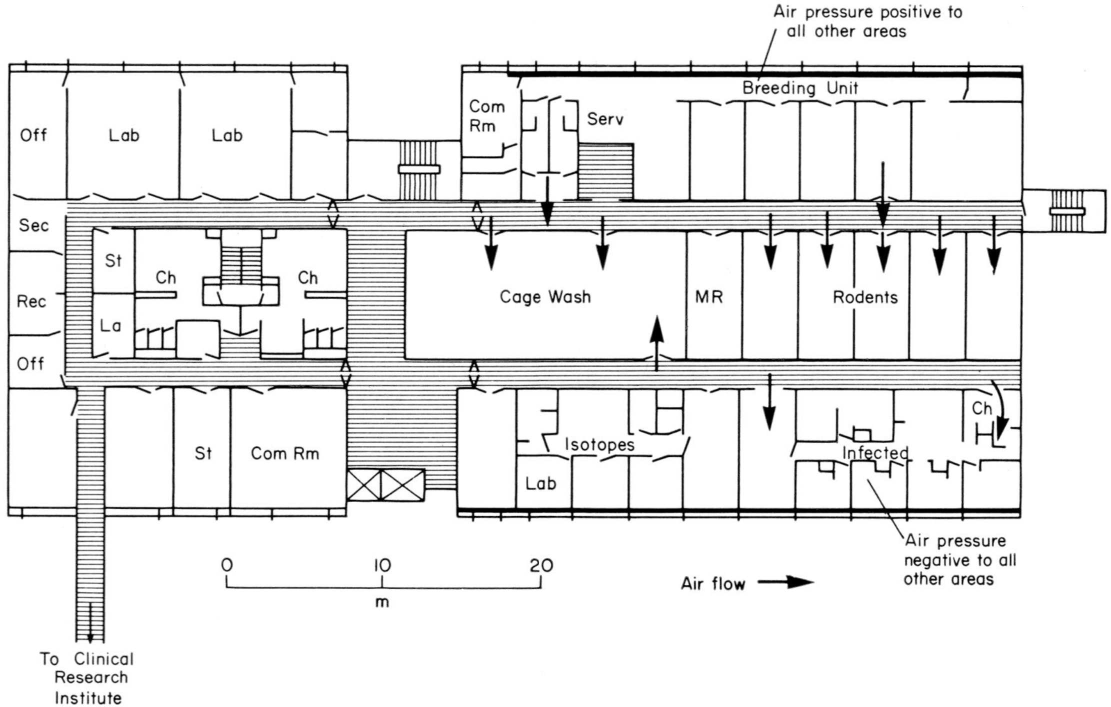

Off, Office
Lab, Laboratory
Rec/Sec, Reception
St, Store
MR, Manipulation Room

La, Laundry
Ch, Changing Room
Com Rm, Common Room
Serv, Service Area

Appendix 3

Level 2

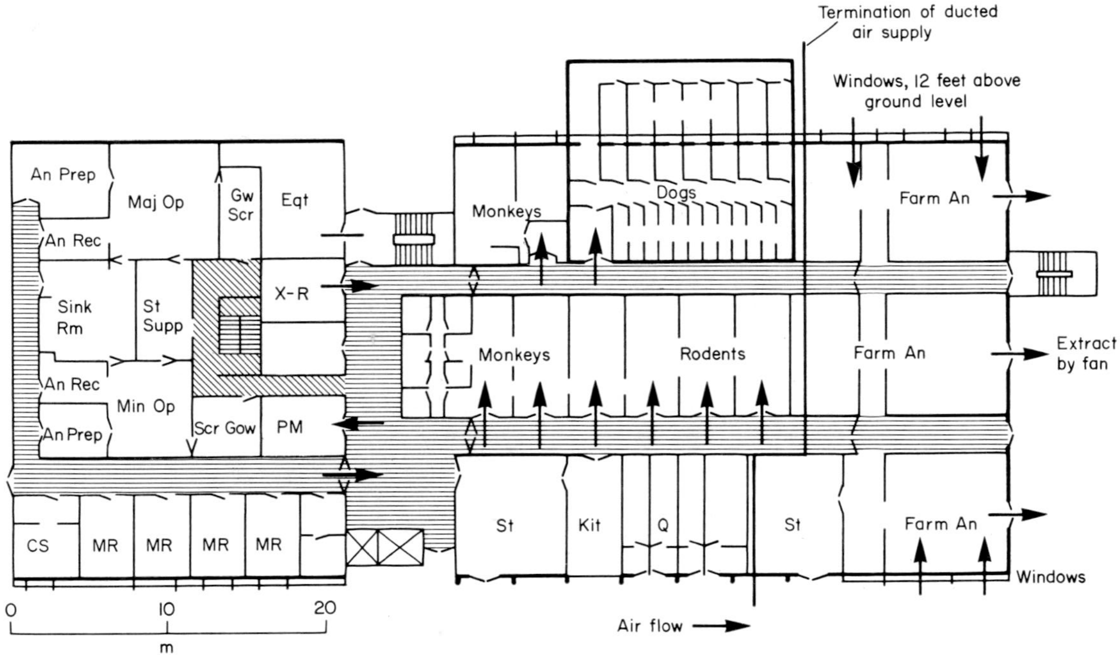

An Prep, Animal Preparation
An Rec, Animal Recovery
Sink Rm, Preparation Room
St Supp, Sterile Supply
Maj Op, Major Operating Theatre

Min Op, Minor Operating Theatre
CS, Cobalt Source
PM, *Post Mortem* Room
EQT/X-R, X-Ray Rooms
Gw Scr, Scrub Rooms

St, Store
Kit, Food Preparation
Q, Isolation Rooms
MR, Manipulation Rooms

Subject Index

V

W